Treatment of Functional Seizures

in Children and Adolescents

A Mind-Body Manual for Health Professionals

Blanche Savage, Catherine Chudleigh,
Clare Hawkes, Stephen Scher, Kasia Kozlowska

AUSTRALIANACADEMIC**PRESS**

First published 2022 by:
Australian Academic Press Group Pty. Ltd.
Samford Valley QLD, Australia
www.australianacademicpress.com.au

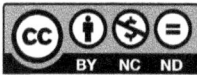

A catalogue record for this
book is available from the
National Library of Australia

ISBN   978-1-925644-61-6   (ebook)
ISBN   978-1-925644-62-3   (paperback)

Disclaimer

Every effort has been made in preparing this work to provide information based on accepted standards and practice at the time of publication. The publisher and author, however, make no representations or warranties with respect to the accuracy or completeness of the contents of this book and specifically disclaim any implied warranties of merchantability or fitness for a particular purpose. It is sold on the understanding that the publisher is not engaged in rendering professional services and neither the publisher nor the author shall be liable for damages arising herefrom. If professional advice or other expert assistance is required, the services of a competent professional should be sought.

Publisher & Editor: Stephen May
Cover design: Luke Harris, Working Type Studio
Typesetting: Australian Academic Press
Printing: Lightning Source

Really practical treatment manuals for functional neurological disorder — with sufficient detail to help clinicians treat their patients — are an urgent need. That is why this wonderful new resource from Blanche Savage, Kasia Kozlowska, and their team in Sydney will be so useful to any health professional seeing people with functional seizures and their families. The manual has been devised for children and young people, but I will be sharing it with therapists who work with adults. It is brimming with practical tips, case examples, and hope for people with functional seizures. Functional neurological disorder is a condition where the whole team need to understand a bit of what everyone can offer, which is why I will also be sharing with neurologists, trainees, and with interested patients and families, too.

Professor Jon Stone
Consultant Neurologist (NHS Lothian)
Honorary Professor (University of Edinburgh)
Department of Clinical Neurosciences
Edinburgh, Scotland

The medical management of paediatric functional neurological disorders can be truly complex and challenging. This detailed new resource by long-experienced clinicians should therefore be a godsend not just for paediatricians and neurologists but, importantly, for paediatric liaison child psychiatrists, psychologists, and their teams, working with cases such as these at the interface between physical and mental health. The emphasis on the contribution of stress and on its biological and psychological underpinnings is a particularly welcome and important contribution. The manual fills a void in the literature and will reward careful reading because of the wealth of insights, the richness of the therapeutic detail, and the vivid vignettes that bring the issues to life. It should help empower clinicians and support the development of paediatric/mental health liaison services in this neglected service area.

M Elena Garralda, MD, MPhil, FRCPsych, FRCPCH
Emeritus Professor of Child and Adolescent Psychiatry,
Imperial College London, England

The Mind-Body Team from The Children's Hospital at Westmead should be acknowledged for this wonderful manual, which constitutes a very useful guideline for managing young people with functional seizures. It is impressive to see how the team translate their extensive clinical expertise and up-to-date research into comprehensive yet easily understandable principles for treating the disorder, illustrated by inspiring case examples. The central 'Stress-System Model' can be flexible and used according to the needs of the young person and families as well as the skills of the clinicians. It successfully bridges the unhelpful mind-body dualism which so often leads to misconceptions about functional seizures. Thus this manual could also be a huge step towards resolving the prejudices and stigmatisation that these families are sadly still experiencing both within and outside the health care system. I gladly recommend its use for all therapists and clinicians working in this field — across English- and non-English-speaking countries.

Charlotte Ulrikka Rask, MD, PhD
Consultant and Clinical Professor, Team for Functional Disorders
Department of Child and Adolescent Psychiatry
Aarhus University Hospital – Psychiatry
Department of Clinical Medicine
Aarhus University, Aarhus, Denmark

This comprehensive and practical treatment approach for children and adolescents with functional seizures reflects the clinical wisdom and research experience of the Mind-Body Team from The Children's Hospital at Westmead that has been developed over many decades. This easy-to-read book takes the practitioner through the process of making and delivering a diagnosis of functional seizures before outlining a flexible and sensible treatment plan based on the Stress-System Model. The authors have done a superb job of integrating the biopsychosocial model with a developmental and family system–based approach. Rich clinical case examples will help even the novice clinician feel comfortable managing this common yet disabling disorder in the outpatient setting. This book should be a core text for any mental health professional working with patients with functional somatic complaints.

Richard J. Shaw, MD
Professor of Psychiatry and Pediatrics
Stanford University School of Medicine
Palo Alto, California, USA

This open access publication has been generously supported by the Estate of the Late A.H. and M.J. Sims of New South Wales, Australia through The Westmead Institute for Medical Research. 'Bert' and 'Joan' were much-loved parents, grandparents, and great-grandparents who enjoyed travelling and meeting new people. They were well known in their community as small businesspeople who supported many community and charitable organisations. Six decades ago, Bert and Joan struggled to bring questions regarding their own young daughter's neurological disorder to the attention of health professionals. Those questions were never answered. It was their wish to improve accessibility to effective health care for children and parents while simultaneously supporting health professionals and medical researchers. This is precisely what this manual achieves. We honour Bert and Joan for their thoughtful generosity, and their family for supporting this valuable publication, knowing it will help clinicians around the world to provide more compassionate and effective care to children with functional seizures, a subtype of functional neurological disorder.

This practical and scholarly manual on the treatment of functional seizures in children and adolescents is astutely written by five leaders in the field: Blanche Savage, Catherine Chudleigh, Clare Hawkes, Stephen Scher, and Kasia Kozlowska. As background, functional neurological disorder (FND) and the related spectrum of functional somatic symptoms are commonly encountered by pediatricians, internists, neurologists, psychiatrists, psychologists, allied mental health providers, and rehabilitation specialists. Functional seizures, a highly prevalent subtype of FND, manifest as acute-onset events that grossly resemble epileptic seizures — yet symptoms are not driven by epileptiform neural activity but rather reflect a problem of brain network function occurring in the context of a nuanced interplay between biological, psychological, and sociocultural factors. Individuals with functional seizures frequently utilize health care resources across emergency department, acute inpatient, and outpatient clinical settings. While historically neglected as a borderland condition at the intersection of neurology, psychiatry, and psychology, interest in functional seizures and FND more broadly has, thankfully, increased greatly over the past several decades. Nonetheless, many health care providers lack expertise in managing children and adolescents with functional seizures and other functional symptoms — an important gap that is addressed by this manual.

Within an integrated (and forward-thinking) brain-mind-body framework, this book provides health care professionals with an invaluable guide on how to treat paediatric functional seizures. The book begins with a chapter on the *rule-in* approach to functional seizures, leveraging clinical history, neurological features, and adjunctive video-electroencephalography data. The biopsychosocial formulation, critical to the development of a patient-centered treatment plan, is subsequently highlighted. Education of children and adolescents with functional seizures, their family members, and their extended networks can be considered an important aspect of initial treatment. In my opinion, the chapter on 'The Five-Step Plan for Managing Functional Seizures' is a major highlight of this book – with the metaphor of 'surfing the wave' having broad appeal. Subsequent psychotherapy-focused chapters detail a therapeutic approach that leverages 'bottom-up' as well as 'top-down' mind-body principles to promote recovery. This material is followed by an important chapter in how to effectively manage co-occurring mental health concerns. Toward the end of the book, chapters underscore the utility of team-based care, practically describing how to effectively partner with the family, the school, and the medical team.

In summary, this is a timely and much-needed book in the field. My hope is that this manual will help to reduce the suffering of children and adolescents experiencing functional seizures by growing the number of clinicians who feel well equipped to care skilfully for this population.

David L. Perez, MD, MMSc
Massachusetts General Hospital
Associate Professor, Harvard Medical School

We begin by acknowledging our fundamental debt to Dr Kenneth Nunn, a child and adolescent psychiatrist who, way back in 1994, had the foresight to develop an inpatient rehabilitation program — now known as the Mind-Body Program — for children (including adolescents) with functional somatic symptoms at The Royal Alexandra Children's Hospital (now renamed The Children's Hospital at Westmead). At that time, Dr Nunn also established functional neurological (conversion) disorder as a bona fide neuropsychiatric disorder (Nunn, 1998) — two decades earlier than the disorder came to be accepted in the broader literature (Perez et al., 2021). Working alongside Dr Nunn from the inception of the rehabilitation program, through to the establishment of the Mind-Body Program, and continuing until her retirement in 2013, was Sister Margaret English. Initially the nursing unit manager of Hall Ward, the paediatric ward (much later, a psychiatric ward) to which Dr Nunn's patients were admitted, Sister Margaret subsequently moved into the role of clinical nursing consultant (CNC) in Psychological Medicine.

Next, we acknowledge Prof Leanne Williams a neuroscientist who — alongside Drs Kerrie Brown, Loyola McLean, and Angie Claussen – took the last author, Dr Kasia Kozlowska, under her wing as one of her PhD students. In 2006, Prof Williams was director of the Brain Dynamics Centre at The Westmead Institute of Medical Research (WIMR). The PhD project involved the setting up of a paediatric FND research program at WIMR that continues to this day. Close links were forged, and when Prof Williams took up a position at Stanford University, the collaboration between the mind-body team and researchers at WIMR's Brain Dynamics Centre — Drs Mayuresh Korgaonkar, Kristi Griffiths, and Isabella Breukelaar — continued.

We thank all the children and adolescents — those with functional neurological disorder (including functional seizures), as well as controls — who participated in the different studies within our research program at WIMR. These studies, alongside the work done by colleagues all around the world, have provided our mind-body team with an evidence base that we have progressively refined and used to update the treatment components that make up our Mind-Body Program. This evidence base also informs the treatment interventions described in this manual (see Appendix A).

At The Children's Hospital at Westmead, many other clinicians, departments, and administrators have supported our work treating children with functional seizures in the Mind-Body Program. Here we begin by mentioning our hospital administrators, who have recognized both the clinical value of that work and its potential contribution to the broader field of psychological medicine. In this context we give particular thanks to Christie Breen, Catherine Cruz, Katherine Knight, and Andrea Worth. We also acknowledge the bed managers from our hospital, who have worked hard over the years to make beds available for our patients with functional seizures (and functional neurological disorder more generally); our neurology colleagues, including the nursing staff and EEG technicians, from Commercial Travellers Ward and the TY Nelson Department of Neurology and Neurosurgery, who make the process of diagnosis and referral appear seamless; the nursing staff on Wade Ward, a therapeutic adolescent ward, whose patience, kindness, and clinical skills never cease to amaze us; the physiotherapy staff, who help our patients build physical and emotional resilience, and who manage their functional seizures with practiced calm; and the teaching staff from the hospital school, who welcome the children into their class and provide them with the assurance and confidence that they need in order to manage the classroom setting.

We are grateful for the enthusiasm, encouragement, and good will of the numerous health care professionals who read our draft chapters and gave us such helpful feedback. From David Perez's Functional Neurological Disorder Unit at Massachusetts General Hospital, we thank Daniel Millstein, Sara Finkelstein, and David himself. From the Functional/Dissociative Seizure Task Force of the International League Against Epilepsy, we thank Coraline Hingray and Mercedes Sarudiansky for providing feedback about our Fact Sheet (see Appendix B). We also thank our child and adolescent psychiatry colleagues Helene Helgeland and Kenneth Nunn, our pharmacy colleague Judy Longworth, and our paediatrician colleague — a paediatrician-in-training — Mushira Che Mokhtar. Danae Laskowski, a Child and Adolescent Mental Health Services (CAHMS) clinician, reviewed the draft manual from the perspective of clinicians working in remote rural areas across Australia. Staff from our hospital school and the New South Wales Education Department — Trish Boss, Helen Dawson, Wendy Griffiths, Pauline Kotselas, and Mercedes Wilkinson — provided invaluable assistance in framing the chapter about working with the school. And we owe a debt of gratitude to our registrars Chun Wang Jason Lao, Emily Le Fevre, Yu-Na Kim, Natalie Yuen-Lee Lim, and Joseph Elkadi, who generously supported the author team — in many different ways — while we were writing this manual.

The figures and text boxes in this manual reflect a network of collaborations. We are grateful to Maryllor De and Sister Veronika Chandler for their help with this manual's many illustrations. We thank Danae Laskowski for working with us to modify her Traffic Light Safety Plan for use with functional seizures (see Chapter 6 and Appendix F). We thank Gretel Butler for her help in supporting our team in the use of sensory tools for the treatment of children with functional seizures (see Chapter 7). We thank Clare Harb for her help with the epileptic component of the seizure management plan (see Chapter 14). And we thank Kenneth Nunn and Judy Longworth for their help with the illustration for the medication chapter (see Chapter 15).

At the time of publication, the following colleagues had contributed translations of the book's Fact Sheet and the Five-Step Plan into their native languages. These translations will vastly enhance the capacity of clinicians to discuss functional seizures with children and families from non-English-speaking countries and to engage them constructively in treatment. We are enormous grateful to these translators/colleagues.

Arabic	Zainab Al-Wardi and Dina Mahmood
Chinese (Mandarin)	Velda Han, Jeremy Bingyuan Lin, and Furene Wang
Danish	Karen Hansen Kallesøe, Anne Sofie Hansen, Malene Skjøth, Helle Veller Mortensen, and Charlotte Ulrikka Rask
Finnish	Airi Hautamäki and Milla Syrjänen
French	Pascal Carrive and Coraline Hingray
German	Alexander Lehn
Greek	Harry Field
Hebrew	Sharon Barak, Etzyona Eisenstein, Maya Gerner, Jana Landa, and Tamar Silberg
Hindi	Vinita Bansal, Rachita Narang, and Nidhi Purohit
Italian	Giangennaro Coppola, Francesca Operto, and Grazia Pastorino
Japanese	Kenichi Mikami
Kurdish	Hozan Ali
Lithuanian	Miglė Marcinkevičiūtė and Danutė Gailienė
Norwegian	Helene Helgeland and Kine Krohg
Persian	Maryam Homayoun
Polish	Alicja Kozlowska, Daniela Kozlowska, and Anna Szaflarska-Poplawska
Portuguese	Rui Ferreira Carvalho, Carla Maia, Inês Pinto, and Rui Pires Sampaio
Russian	Svetlana Klimanova and Natalia Pleshkova
Spanish	Mercedes Sarudiansky and Camila Wolfzun
Swahili	Eddie Chengo
Ukrainian	Alexander Saksonov

Our paediatric colleagues, here in Australia and also abroad, who diagnose or treat functional seizures — Russell Dale, Leon Dure, Aaron Fobian, Shekeeb Mohammad, Tyson Sawchuk, Areti Vassilopoulos, and Jeff Waugh — have been a constant source not only of invaluable insights drawn from their own work and thinking, but of inspiration and support. We thank Alan Carson and Jon Stone for paving the way for others through their groundbreaking work with adults and their efforts to develop user-friendly resources for clinicians (see, e.g., Carson and colleagues [2015]).

The manual includes many stories of lived experience. We thank those children and adolescents — and their families — who gave us consent to share their stories because they wanted to be able to help others. We thank Bernadette (pseudonym) for sharing her reflections of the therapeutic process in the last chapter (Chapter 16). The other stories in this manual are amalgams drawn from our experience of similar cases.

We also thank our editor Stephen May for making space for this manual among his press's publications for 2022 and for his flexibility both in adjusting to the demands of publishing this manual open access and in enabling us to make various resources available online. The knowledge that Australian Academic Press had a home for this manual, coupled with Stephen's quiet confidence that we would bring this project to fruition, provided us with a sense of grounding throughout the writing process.

Carson, A., Lehn, A., Ludwig, L., & Stone, J. (2015). Explaining functional disorders in the neurology clinic: A photo story. *Pract Neurol, 16*(1), 56–61. https://doi.org/10.1136/practneurol-2015-001242

Nunn, K. (1998). Neuropsychiatry in childhood: residential treatment. In J. Green & B. Jacobs (Eds.), *In-patient child psychiatry: Modern practice, research and the future* (pp. 259–283). Jessica Kingsley.

Perez, D. L., Edwards, M. J., Nielsen, G., Kozlowska, K., Hallett, M., & LaFrance, W. C., Jr. (2021). Decade of progress in motor functional neurological disorder: Continuing the momentum. *J Neurol Neurosurg Psychiatry, 16*, 668–677. https://doi.org/10.1136/jnnp-2020-323953

Blanche Savage

Blanche Savage, a clinical psychologist, has been a core member of the mind-body, consultation-liaison team at The Children's Hospital at Westmead for 13 years. On joining the team, her first patient was an adolescent girl presenting with functional seizures in the context of a difficult family situation. It marked the beginning of what has become a deep, long-standing interest in children and adolescents with functional somatic symptoms, including functional seizures, and how to help them return to health and wellbeing. The current manual is an effort to share what the team has learned with other clinicians around the world. One of the interventions that Blanche uses extensively in her own work is hypnosis. Along with Helene Helgeland and Kasia Kozlowska, she has contributed a chapter — 'Hypnosis in the Treatment of Functional Somatic Symptoms in Children and Adolescents' — to the *Routledge International Handbook of Clinical Hypnosis*, to be published early in 2023.

Catherine Chudleigh

Catherine Chudleigh, a clinical psychologist, has been a core member of the mind-body, consultation-liaison team at The Children's Hospital at Westmead for 12 years. Alongside other clinicians in the team, she has helped to develop a range of child-friendly interventions for children and adolescents with functional somatic symptoms (including functional seizures). She has a particular interest in helping her patients to become aware of body states and to manage states of high arousal. In this context she has used heart rate variability to support children's awareness of their emotional and physiological state and also as a means of tracking their treatment response to calming interventions. This use of heart rate variability is highlighted in a forthcoming 2023 publication, *Implementing Evidence-Based Mind-Body Interventions for Children and Adolescents with Functional Neurological Disorder* (Kasia Kozlowska, Catherine Chudleigh, and other team members) with the *Harvard Review of Psychiatry*.

Clare Hawkes

Clare Hawkes, a clinical psychologist, has been a core member of the mind-body, consultation-liaison team at The Children's Hospital at Westmead for two years. Clare brings energy and initiative to the mind-body team. She particularly enjoys the interface between medicine and psychological work. Clare utilises a wide variety of sensory strategies as calming interventions. She also has a special interest in neuropsychology assessments, and she conducts these assessments for young people in the Mind-Body Program who have difficulties in learning or other neurodevelopment concerns. She has taken on important role in the mind-body team's neuromodulation study (with the Safe and Sound protocol) and, in that context, was a co-author of a recent case study published in the *Harvard Review of Psychiatry*. She is currently completing a Masters in Clinical Neuropsychology to build upon and extend this skill set.

Stephen Scher

Stephen Scher taught clinical medical ethics in Harvard Medical School–affiliated hospitals in the 1980s, spent several years at Yale Law School and Yale School of Management (teaching professional ethics and organizational behavior) in the 1990s, and joined the editorial staff of the *American Journal of International Law* in 1999 and the editorial staff of the *Harvard Review of Psychiatry* in 2003. At the end of 2016, he stepped down as Senior Editor of the *American Journal*. He is now in his twentieth year as Senior Editor of the *Harvard Review*. His recent publications, both published open access with Palgrave Macmillan, include *Rethinking Health Care Ethics* (2018, with Kasia Kozlowska) and *Functional Somatic Symptoms in Children and Adolescents: A Stress-System Approach to Assessment and Treatment* (2020, with Kasia Kozlowska and Helene Helgeland). A Lecturer in Psychiatry at Harvard Medical School, he has been collaborating with Kasia Kozlowska and other members of the mind-body team for over a decade.

Kasia Kozlowska

Kasia Kozlowska has gained worldwide prominence as a child and adolescent psychiatrist at The Children's Hospital at Westmead, as Clinical Associate Professor at the University of Sydney Medical School, and as Associate Professor and Research Fellow at the Westmead Institute of Medical Research, University of Sydney. In her intertwined clinical and research roles, she heads a multidisciplinary consultation-liaison team, a research program for children with functional neurological disorder, and a program — the Mind-Body Program — for the treatment of children disabled by functional neurological symptoms. She and her team are committed to the close integration of research findings and clinical practice, and to making the products of their clinical work and research broadly available to other professionals. Her 2020 open access book, *Functional Somatic Symptoms in Children and Adolescents: A Stress-System Approach to Assessment and Treatment*, is a free resource available to clinicians, as are many of her clinical and research publications.

Contents

Appendix C

Appendix D

Appendix E

Appendix F1

Appendix F2

Appendix G

Chapter 1

Introduction

In this treatment manual for functional seizures in children, adolescents, and young adults — 'young people' — we present the program developed by the mind-body team at The Children's Hospital at Westmead, a tertiary care paediatric hospital located in New South Wales, Australia. The team's Mind-Body Program, organised as part of a consultation-liaison psychiatry service within the Department of Psychological Medicine, works with young people, up to the age of 18 years, who present with functional somatic symptoms, including functional seizures. This manual describes the treatment interventions we have developed over the last 20 years through clinical trial and error, by translating research findings into our clinical practice, and by evaluating our own treatment interventions through prospective cohort studies. This treatment manual uses the Stress-System Model for functional somatic symptoms, elaborated in *Functional Somatic Symptoms in Children and Adolescents: A Stress-System Approach to Assessment and Treatment* (Kozlowska, Scher, & Helgeland, 2020) — available open access (see reference list). We believe that it would be helpful for clinicians to acquaint themselves with the model (see especially Chapter 4) before using the manual.

The goal of this treatment program for functional seizures is for young people to return to good health and to normal functioning and wellbeing. Treatment outcomes for young people who follow this treatment program are very positive, and our expectation is that a young person with functional seizures who follows the program will experience major clinical improvement (Vassilopoulos et al., 2022).

The Different Names That Clinicians Use for Functional Seizures

Across the history of medicine, functional seizures have been called by many different names. The most common names still used today include *psychogenic non-epileptic seizures*, *stress seizures*, and *dissociative seizures*. Opinions still vary as to the best terminology (Wardrope et al., 2021). For a discussion of terminology and a list of synonyms, see Chapter 4 and Figure 4.2.

In this manual we use the term *functional seizures* for consistency. Functional seizures are a subtype of functional neurological disorder (FND).[1] *Functional neurological disorder* is the umbrella term for the full range of functional neurological symptoms that present in clinical practice (see Figure 1.1). Functional motor symptoms and functional seizures are the two most common presentations.

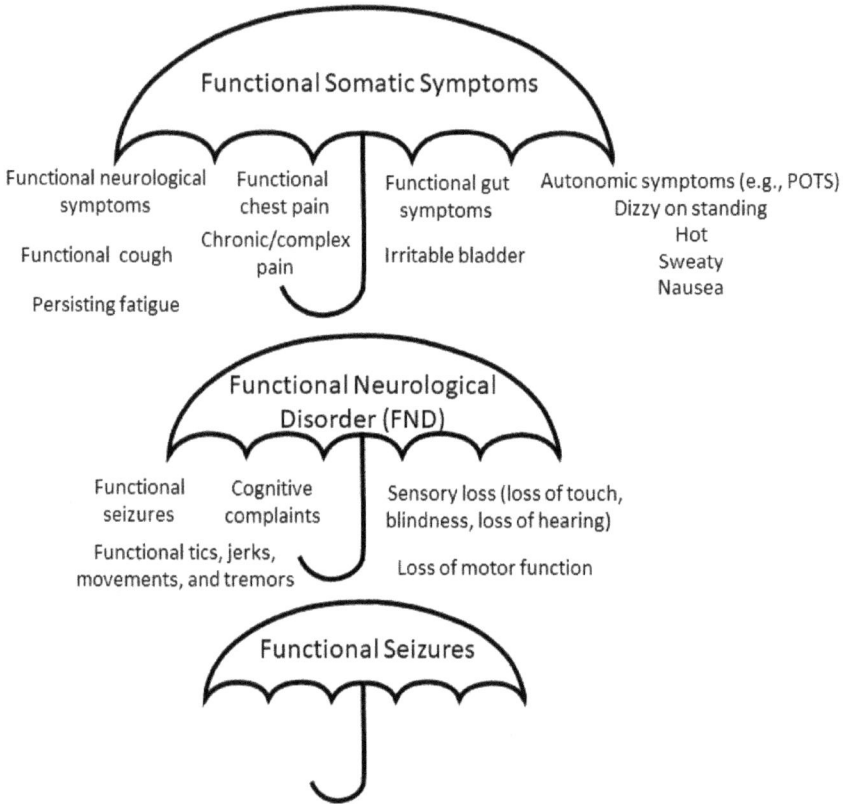

Figure 1.1 Symptoms falling under the umbrella of functional somatic symptoms. Visual presentation showing that functional seizures sit under the umbrella of functional neurological disorder, which, in turn, sits under the broader umbrella of functional somatic symptoms. POTS = postural orthostatic tachycardia syndrome. © Kasia Kozlowska 2019

---

1 In the latest, fifth edition of the *Diagnostic and Statistical Manual of Mental Disorders* (DSM-5), functional neurological disorder is called *functional neurological symptom disorder* (American Psychiatric Association, 2013). Clinicians working in the field, however, use *functional neurological disorder* (FND) because this term has a simplicity and ease of flow.

Functional Seizures Are More Common in Girls and Women

In the civilian (vs. military) setting, functional somatic symptoms occur more frequently in girls and women than in boys and men. Presumably, this difference reflects the impact of female sex hormones not only on stress-system function but also on epigenetics and the modulation of neural networks. To reflect this clinical reality, and for simplicity, we generally use the pronouns *she* and *her* in the present manual. Clinicians working with boys and young men — or with gender-fluid young people — can change the pronouns in their mind's eye to suit their particular clinical milieus.

What Are Functional Seizures?

The brain is a complex biological system made up of neural (brain) networks[2] — clusters of nerves and neural pathways that, in health and wellbeing, work together in balance and synchrony to enable normal motor, sensory, interoceptive, emotional, and cognitive function. In response to the challenges of daily living, these brain and body systems activate, preparing the body for action. And in the normal course of events, after the challenge is met or has passed, arousal then decreases, returning brain and body systems back to baseline.

In young people experiencing serious distress or high arousal, however, this normal balance and synchrony can be lost. The brain and body systems can move into a state of overdrive and temporary dysregulation, potentially resulting in functional seizures, which are sudden, time-limited episodes of neural network dysregulation.

Most young people can sense the approach of a functional seizure because they become aware of the signs and symptoms of activation (increasing brain and body arousal) — a key element of functional seizures. Others learn, with practice, to sense the warning signs of an impending functional seizure.

During the functional seizure itself, the young person typically experiences a loss of voluntary control of motor function, including shaking, jerking, twitching, loss of movement, or falling down (syncope/fainting-like episodes). The young person can also experience a change in consciousness — or even loss of consciousness — including zoning out, cognitive clouding, feeling weird or disconnected, or being unresponsive. Some young people may experience unusual body sensations or various strong emotions, such as weeping, crying out, moaning, or wailing.

---

2 Alternative language for neural networks — when talking to younger children — includes *brain networks*, *brain systems*, or just *the brain*.

When the functional seizure has run its course, the young person should be able to resume normal activities. Feelings of fatigue are common because significant energy has been expended. Headache is common. Occasionally, other functional neurological symptoms may be triggered during the functional seizure — for example, a loss of motor function in some part of the body, such as the legs — and these symptoms may take longer to resolve.

What Is the Difference Between Functional Seizures and Epileptic Seizures?

All seizures occur when the normal balance and synchrony in neural networks have been lost.

Epileptic seizures occur when the balance and synchrony within and between neural networks is temporarily disrupted due to abnormal electrical activity in the brain. This abnormal activity can be identified by the neurologist on electroencephalogram (EEG), a test that measures electrical activity in the brain. The EEG was invented in 1929 — nearly a century ago — by the German doctor Hans Berger. Before that time, the cause of epileptic seizures had not been understood. By contrast, the brain's electrical activity is *not* disrupted in functional seizures.

Because the treatment plans differ radically for epileptic versus functional seizures, determining which is which is a matter of crucial clinical importance.

Many mental health clinicians find it helpful to conceptualise functional seizures, or at least many of them, as a more severe form of panic attack: a state of extreme brain and body arousal. As in a panic attack, the body is excessively activated, which results in sweating, increased heart rate, and hyperventilation. But the arousal is so strong that neural networks reach the limit of their capacity to maintain biological stability, and they become temporarily dysregulated, resulting in the functional seizure. When the functional seizure is over, the neural networks reset themselves, and normal function is restored.

For a brief summary of the current research — the knowledge base that underpins our current understanding and our current working hypothesis — see Appendix A.

In young people, a broad range of physical, psychological, relational, and academic stressors — especially when cumulative, repetitive, chronic, or overwhelming, resulting in a state of sustained arousal — can cause neural networks to become overactive and dysregulated.

- Physical stressors, such as pain, fatigue, and illness (e.g., viral infection, minor injury, or medical procedures)

- Psychological stressors, such as thoughts or images of distressing past events, thoughts or images predicting negative future events, and strong negative emotions[3] (anxiety, fear, anger, distress)

- Relational stressors, such as conflict in the family, grief and loss, and friendship issues (including bullying and social exclusion)

- Academic stressors, such as high expectations of academic achievement, or academic problems in the context of learning difficulties

- Stressors associated with competitive sports (e.g., pushing oneself too hard)

- Less commonly, high levels of excitement, pleasure, or physical activity, generating high states of arousal.

Why Are Some Children and Young People Vulnerable to Functional Seizures?

In thinking about functional seizures clinicians need to use a biopsychosocial approach. The various biological, psychological, and social factors that predispose young people to functional seizures are the topic of current research. What we do know is that the neurobiology is very complicated. In our work in the mind-body team, we have found that most young people who experience functional seizures have a history of physical, emotional, or interpersonal stress — also known as adverse childhood experiences (ACEs) — and that this stress is often cumulative. Current research highlights that ACEs are biologically embedded in the body and brain, making the body and brain more sensitive and reactive in the face of further life challenges and stress (Boyce et al., 2021; Nelson, 2013). Figure 1.2 provides a visual representation of some of the complex interactions — between different factors — that play a role in the aetiology of functional seizures.

What Is the Stress-System Model?

The Stress-System Model is what we (the authors) and our mind-body team use to think about, understand, and treat functional somatic symptoms (including functional seizures) (see Figure 1.3). Our team developed the model after we

---

3 In this manual we use Antonio Damasio and Gil Carvalho's terminology for emotions and feelings. Emotions refer to neurophysiological changes in body state, and feelings are the subjective experience of those states (Damasio & Carvalho, 2013).

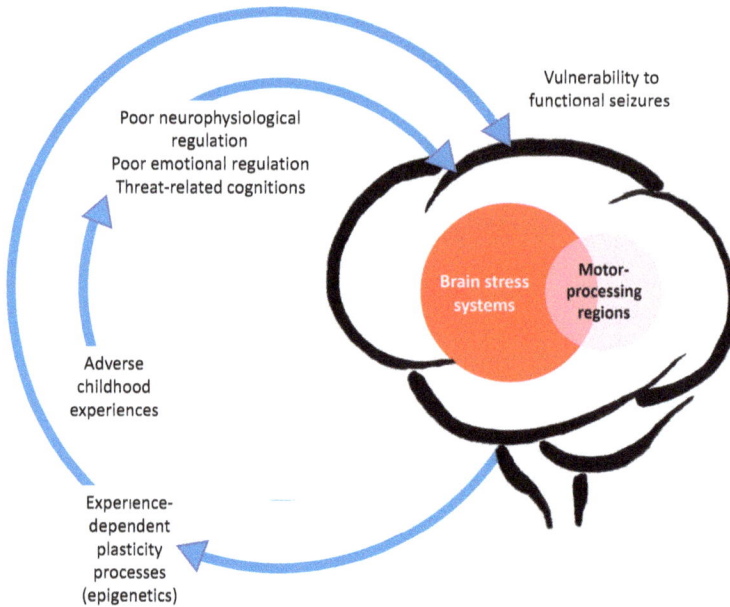

Figure 1.2 The hypothetical aetiology of functional seizures. Visual representation linking adverse life experiences, stress-system activation, and epigenetic/plasticity processes that increase vulnerability for functional seizures (functional neurological disorder). © Kasia Kozlowska 2021

came across the work of George Chrousos — a paediatric endocrinologist and neuroscientist — who, together with colleagues, had introduced the idea of the stress system as a systemic framework for looking at the diverse and interrelated biological systems that underpin stress-related illnesses (Chrousos et al., 1988). The Stress-System Model depicts the different components of the stress system and explains how an overactivated or dysregulated stress system — or a stress system that remains in a state of chronic overactivation — can underpin a broad array of functional somatic symptoms (including functional seizures). Following the Stress-System Model, treatment for functional seizures involves interventions that help down-regulate (calm down) the stress system and that facilitate balance and synchrony within brain networks and within and between body systems.

In discussing the stress system, we sometimes refer to the stress system as a whole (*stress system*) and sometimes to subsystem components (*stress systems*) that make up the stress system (see Figure 1.3).

Functional Seizures, Arousal, and the Regulation of Energy

Young people with functional seizures typically experience a state of increasing arousal — and activation of body systems — prior to their functional seizures

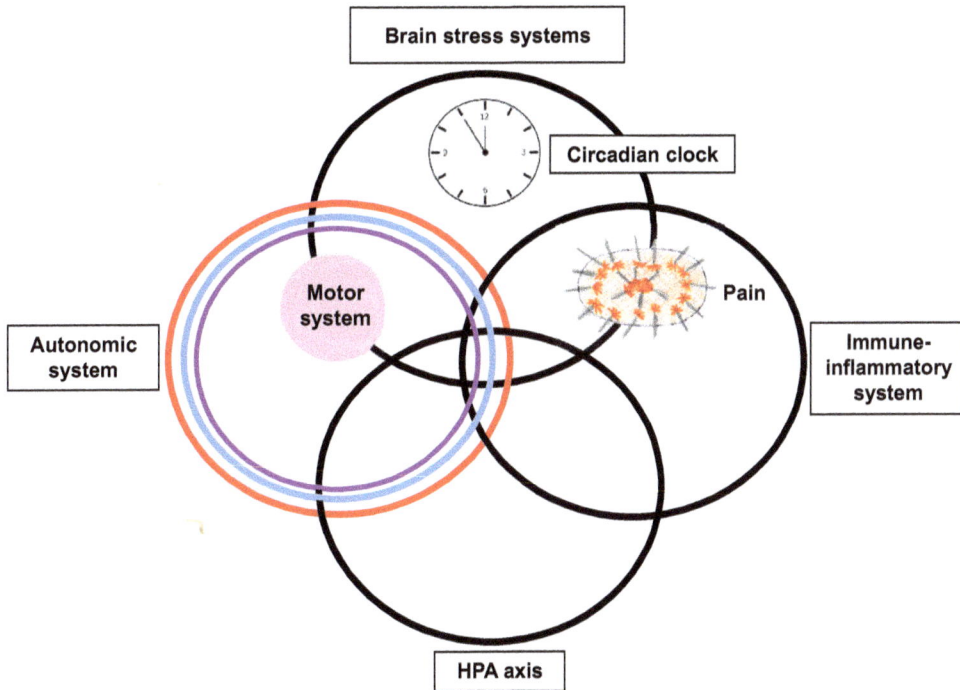

Figure 1.3 The stress-system model for functional somatic symptoms: Circles metaphor. The overlap between the different components of the stress system — the hypothalamic-pituitary-adrenal axis, autonomic nervous system, immune-inflammatory system, and brain stress systems — is presented by the overlap between the circles. HPA = hypothalamic-pituitary-adrenal. © Kasia Kozlowska 2013

(see also Chapter 4). This activation, of necessity, requires a high use of energy. Regulation of energy use is a core function of the stress system (see Figure 1.3). Stress hormones (the hormonal component of the stress system) and the autonomic nervous system (the neural component) work together to increase the body's capacity for increased energy use.[4]

When an individual experiences her body state as calm wellbeing — a state that optimises the capacity to connect with others — energy use is usually in the midrange: not too high and not too low. When the young person's body state reflects a defensive state — a response to a threat or stressor, real or perceived — energy use typically increases (reflecting high arousal states). If the defensive state is maintained, energy use may remain very high (sustained high arousal), or it may suddenly plummet to levels that are very low (reflecting low arousal [shutdown] states) (Kozlowska, Walker, et al., 2015).

---

4 For more information about the regulation of energy, see Chapters 6 and 8 in Kozlowska, Scher, and Helgeland (2020).

Research studies suggest that the issue of energy regulation is of particular relevance to functional seizures. EEG studies with children and adolescents with functional seizures (vs. healthy controls) show increased activation of neural networks in the resting state and in response to hyperventilation (Braun et al., 2021; Radmanesh et al., 2020). A pilot study of brain temperature in three adult patients with functional seizures showed increased brain temperatures, presumably reflecting activation of the stress system and of neural networks underpinning neurophysiological and emotion regulation, coupled with high energy use (Sharma & Szaflarski, 2021). One current hypothesis about the underlying cause of functional seizures is that neural networks become unstable when experiencing strong perturbations in energy flow, including the additional demands for energy in the context of new threats or stressors, perceived or real (Radmanesh et al., 2020). Put simply, neural networks may dysregulate when energy demands exceed biological limits. The result is a functional seizure.

How to Use This Manual

In our own inpatient hospital setting, the treatment interventions described in this manual are delivered by a multidisciplinary team using a multimodal approach — where different members of the consultation-liaison team contribute different elements of the treatment. Likewise, the arrangement or choice of interventions in this manual is presented in the order that our mind-body team typically delivers them. But because the range of issues that young people bring to therapy may differ widely, the order of the therapeutic interventions sometimes needs to be changed — tailored to match the needs and capacities of each patient and family.

Therapists and other clinicians will need to adapt the ideas presented in this manual to their own specific clinical contexts — public or private; inpatient, day program, or outpatient; team based or solo practitioner working alongside other professionals in the community — and also to the particular needs of the young people and families that they see. We want to highlight that the manual is intended only as a general template to be flexibly implemented, taking into account not just the needs of patients and families but the particular capacities and skills of the therapists and other clinicians providing the treatment. We assume, moreover, that the interventions and the order of the interventions should be guided by a biopsychosocial formulation for each case — that is, by a synthesis or coherent summary of the relevant factors that contribute to each young person's presentation (Gordon et al., 2005; Henderson & Martin, 2014; Winters et al., 2007). It is important to note that this manual is not designed as a self-help guide for patients or families to use independently without the support of a therapist or clinician.

Although learning to care for and treat young people with functional seizures may initially appear a daunting task, you need to recognise that, as mental health clinicians, your training and your skill sets already provide you with most of the tools needed to work with these patients. That said, in the process of reading through this manual, you will need to think carefully about your existing tools, carefully determine which elements will help you with this particular patient population, and identify what additions or changes might be required for you — given your current skills and knowledge — to address the needs of these patients. You may find is that this process requires some relearning.

As a final observation, though we refer to the present work as a *manual*, it does not set forth what might be considered *manualised* treatment or therapy. Just the reverse is true. What we provide are general guidelines, methods, and insights that clinicians need to keep in mind as they approach the care of each individual patient in this diverse patient population. Each patient is different, and the *care* of each patient needs to be different. There will, to be sure, be recognisable patterns in providing such care — patterns that we have attempted to describe in this manual — but the particular shape of each young person's care will, of necessity, depend upon and reflect the knowledge, skills, and creativity of each particular clinician.

Chapter 2

The Diagnosis of Functional Seizures by the Paediatric Neurologist

It is important for mental health clinicians who treat functional seizures to understand the medical process by which functional seizures are diagnosed. This knowledge enables the clinician to ensure that the following elements of the medical assessment have been completed:

- The young person has had appropriate medical consultations and investigations.

- The young person has been given a positive diagnosis of functional seizures.

- The young person (and her family)[1] has been given an explanation about functional seizures from the neurologist or the paediatrician.

- The young person (and her family) has accepted the diagnosis and agreed to proceed with a mind-body intervention with the mental health clinician.

The Medical Process for Assessing Functional Seizures

Functional seizures are best assessed by a paediatric neurologist who has clinical expertise in functional seizures. The neurologist makes the diagnosis based on clinical history, descriptions by witnesses, home videos, and video encephalogram (vEEG). vEEG is the gold standard assessment for the diagnosis of functional seizures (Tatum et al., 2022; Whitehead et al., 2017). It shows that the functional seizures are not accompanied by a spike-and-wave pattern, which is the signature pattern of epileptic seizures.

---

1 As noted in Chapter 1, because functional somatic symptoms occur more frequently in girls than in boys, we generally use the pronouns *she* and *her* to reflect this clinical reality.

In some clinical settings the vEEG may not be available or may be available only after a long wait. In that case, the diagnosis can be made with an EEG (which will show no seizure activity) and evaluation of home videos by a paediatric neurologist who sees functional seizures frequently and is skilled in identifying clinical features common to functional seizures.

In Australia, where it can be hard to access such specialists outside of major cities, the young person's family should discuss referral options with their paediatrician (or family doctor). A number of paediatric neurologists are currently offering telehealth consults and may be able to assess home videos of the young person's events remotely (assuming a standard EEG is also available), thereby supporting the local paediatrician (or family doctor) in making a diagnosis. If a paediatric neurologist is unavailable, the referral may need to go to an adult neurologist, who can work with the paediatrician or family doctor to reach a diagnosis.

Providing the Young Person and Family with a Positive Diagnosis, Explanation of the Diagnosis, and Explanation About the Treatment Required

A positive diagnosis of functional seizures provides clear communication and clarity about the young person's medical condition and gives that condition a name (see Text Box 2.1). Statements such as 'your child might have functional seizures [or synonymous term]', 'there is no medical cause', 'it's not epilepsy', or 'it's behavioural' are inadequate. The neurologist or paediatrician also needs to explain the diagnosis and to provide the young person and family with information about the treatment required. More information about this process is available in a book chapter dedicated to this topic (Kozlowska & Mohammad, 2022).

The Appropriate Medical Processes Need to Have Taken Place to Keep Everyone Safe

As mentioned above, the mental health clinician needs to ensure that the appropriate medical assessment processes have taken place:

- *Scope of practice.* Unlike the neurologist, the mental health clinician does not have the clinical skills or investigation tools to make a diagnosis of functional seizures; the necessary medical process is outside of the clinician's scope of practice. For this very reason, the responsibility of making the diagnosis lies with the neurologist or paediatrician and not with the mental health clinician.

Text Box 2.1
Providing a Positive Diagnosis of Functional Seizures

The neurologist's narrative might go something like this:

We have now concluded the neurological assessment. We have completed the physical assessment, a blood panel, and the video EEG. I have looked carefully at the video EEG and also at the video material you provided. I have very good news. The video EEG is normal. This means that [patient's name] does not have epilepsy. The seizures that [patient's name] suffers from are called *functional seizures*. Functional seizures are a subtype of functional neurological disorder. They are very common. We see one to two new patients a week. Functional seizures are unpleasant to experience and to watch, but they are not dangerous.

Are you following me? Do you have any questions?

There has been a lot of research into functional seizures in the last ten years. Our current understanding is that functional seizures reflect a temporary disruption of brain networks. This disruption appears to be triggered by physical or psychological stress. Common physical stress triggers include pain, injuries, or viral illness. Common psychological stress triggers include friendship difficulties, stress from academic work or competitive sports, or conflict in the family. Any of these stress events can activate and dysregulate neural networks.

Are you following me? Do you have any questions?

Functional seizures require prompt treatment. With prompt treatment most young people are able to return to full health. Treatment involves interventions that address the triggers and that help calm the brain. In this hospital, the mind-body team that works in Psychological Medicine specialises in the treatment of functional seizures. I will make a referral. The team will meet with you, do an assessment, and work out a treatment program for [patient's name].

Do you have any questions?

- *Creation of a safe therapeutic context.* The mental health clinician needs the neurologist, paediatrician, or family doctor to make an accurate positive diagnosis to ensure safety for the young person, both medically and in the therapeutic space where the mental health clinician and young person will work together. The key issue here is that functional seizures require mind-body treatment (typically provided by mental health professionals), whereas epileptic seizures require medical treatment with anti-epileptic medication. Since uncontrolled epilepsy can be life-threatening or even fatal (in approximately one in a thousand cases), making the correct diagnosis and ensuring that the young person is safe are of the highest importance.

- *Diagnose and treat early.* An early diagnosis that is made soon after the onset of the functional seizures — followed by prompt treatment — is associated with better clinical outcomes. Most young people who are promptly diagnosed and promptly treated return to full health and wellbeing.

When Things Get More Complicated I: The Young Person Has Both Epileptic and Functional Seizures

In some young people the situation is more complicated because the young person has both epileptic and functional seizures. In this scenario it can be helpful to clarify — with the neurologist (and family) — the clinical pattern of the epileptic seizures (which are the same from one event to the next) and the clinical pattern of the functional seizures (which often change from one event to the next and also evolve over time). If the epileptic seizures are well controlled (by medication) and the family is able to tell the seizures apart, then the treatment intervention is straightforward. There is one management plan for the epileptic seizures and one management plan for the functional seizures, and they are run in parallel. If the epileptic seizures are not well controlled, however, or if the family is unable to tell the seizures apart, then the family will need to err on the side of caution and prioritise the epileptic seizure safety plan when any event occurs.

When Things Get More Complicated II: The Young Person Has Functional Seizures Alongside Other Functional Neurological Symptoms

In other young people the situation is more complicated because the young person has functional seizures alongside other functional neurological symptoms (see Figure 1.1). In this scenario the neurologist will need to provide an explanation of the functional seizures and also an explanation of functional neurological disorder more broadly. The Stress-System Model explanation that our mind-body team most commonly uses to discuss functional neurological order in general is provided in Text Box 2.2. Because comorbid motor

---

Text Box 2.2
Explanation of Functional Neurological Disorder by the Neurologist

The neurologist's narrative might go something like this:
> The structure of the brain and nervous system is 'all good'. But function has been disrupted and needs to be normalised again.

Or, using the stress-system model:
> [Said to the young person with functional seizures, leg pain, and leg weakness, and her family]

> Thank you for giving me such a comprehensive account of your story [developmental history]. Here is a simple picture that summarises the current research [show Figure 2.1]. It shows you the brain stress systems[1] — the red ball represents the parts of the brain that activate with stress. The stress can be physical (e.g., a fall or a viral infection) or psychological (e.g., worrying about the family or falling out with friends). When the red ball becomes too big and too strong, it can disrupt brain networks, causing functional (or stress) seizures. And we know, from the story you told us, that [describe stressors if available] have all been activating the red ball. When that happens, it can affect other motor functions (depicted by the pink ball) — in your case, disrupting function in the legs. And the pain that you are experiencing is called complex pain. When the red ball (that is, the brain stress systems) activates, it switches on what we call *pain maps* in the brain. Once switched on, the pain maps are quite tricky to switch off. That is why we call the pain *complex* pain. And as you can see from the diagram, treatment for all these problems involves interventions that will help you settle the red ball so that is can no longer disrupt things.

> Does that make sense to you?

---

symptoms and comorbid pain are most common, the explanation provided here refers to both (see Text Box 2.2 and Figure 2.1). Visual metaphors pertaining to sensory symptoms and to comorbid fatigue are available in Kozlowska, Scher, and Helgeland (2020).

Summary of the Key Message from This Chapter: Establishing the Foundation for Future Work

Clinicians working in psychological services or in a solo practice should not accept referrals for the treatment of functional seizures if the appropriate medical assessment process has not been completed (see Figure 2.2). The

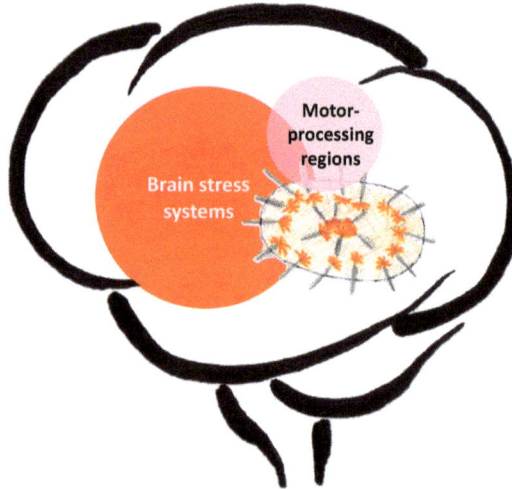

Figure 2.1 Functional neurological disorder involving functional seizures and motor symptoms, with comorbid pain. We use this visual metaphor in explaining functional seizures and functional motor symptoms, with comorbid pain. © Kasia Kozlowska 2019

Tick if completed	Checklist items pertaining to a comprehensive medical assessment
	A comprehensive medical assessment has been completed by a medical practitioner: physical examination, blood panel, and EEG (video EEG or EEG with review of video material by a paediatric neurologist).
	The medical practitioner has provided a positive diagnosis.
	The medical practitioner has provided an explanation.
	The young person and the family understand and accept the diagnosis.

Figure 2.2 Checklist pertaining to a comprehensive medical assessment.

neurologist functions as a gatekeeper: through the medical assessment process, the neurologist creates a safe, secure therapeutic foundation enabling the child, family, and mental health clinician to explore the factors that contributed to the child's presentation.[2]

---

2 See Chapter 2 of Kozlowska, Scher, and Helgeland (2020) for a more in-depth discussion of establishing the secure, safe foundation for future work.

Chapter 3

The Biopsychosocial Assessment: Developing a Biopsychosocial Formulation

The biopsychosocial assessment allows the clinician, the young person, and family to co-construct a formulation — a summary of predisposing, precipitating, and perpetuating factors. This biopsychosocial formulation is used, in turn, to develop a treatment plan and to guide the treatment process. In this chapter we talk to the clinician reader in the first person and share — step by step — the assessment process that our mind-body team follows.

Triage

The assessment and treatment processes described in this manual are appropriate for young people who have already been fully medically investigated and given a positive diagnosis of functional seizures by a medical practitioner — most commonly, a neurologist or paediatrician. As we highlighted in Chapter 2, it is important that the diagnosis be given clearly — for example, 'your child has functional seizures' — and not tentatively or ambiguously. It is also important that all medical investigations be complete, with no relevant results pending. If a new referral meets these criteria, you can proceed with the biopsychosocial assessment. If the referral does not meet these criteria, the referral should be sent back to the young person's medical practitioner, and the process outlined in Chapter 2 should be completed. From the perspective of the neurologist, this process involves the following: the comprehensive medical assessment that supports the diagnosis of functional seizures; communication of the diagnosis; an explanation of the diagnosis; and a general description of the treatment required. From the perspective of the young person and the family, the process involves understanding and accepting the diagnosis of functional seizures.

The Goals of the Initial Assessment

Once you have triaged and accepted the referral, you can begin the biopsychosocial assessment. In our work in the mind-body team, the initial interview always takes place with the family. It involves, at a minimum, both parents and the young person. Because our mind-body team works from a biopsychosocial (systems) perspective, the family interview is not negotiable. If the parents are divorced and amicable, they are both be invited to the assessment; if they are not amicable, then two separate assessments are conducted unless there is a clear reason to exclude one parent (e.g., a history of abuse, estrangement). Stepparents or new partners who live in the family home are also invited to the assessment. The reason for meeting with the young person's family is to help you remain a neutral person in the family system and avoid aligning yourself with any one parent and any one point of view (Rhodes & Wallis, 2011). In our clinical experience, families are also much more likely to be accepting of the formulation and treatment plan when both parents have been included in these discussions from the beginning.

The goals of the initial assessment are as follows:

- To engage the young person and family in the assessment and treatment process

- To briefly understand the family history and background, including a timeline of physical, psychological, and relational stressors (what our mind-body team calls the story of the family and the story of the symptoms)

- To assess for biological markers of physiological dysregulation

- To screen for any potential comorbid mental health condition

- To co-construct a biopsychosocial formulation (a process that typically requires some psychoeducation about functional seizures)

- To negotiate an agreement about the components that will make up the treatment intervention

By the end of the initial interview with the family — through a storytelling process that elicits and helps to shape the story of the young person's developmental history — you and the family should have developed a joint understanding of the functional seizures. This joint understanding is a combination of what the family knows about the young person's presentation and what the clinician knows, and has shared, about functional seizures. The information is formalised into a biopsychosocial formulation, which is articulated aloud in the conversation with the family:

'OK. From what you told me this is how I understand things ...'

The formulation can also be documented visually on a timeline or whiteboard (Helgeland et al., 2022; Førdea et al., 2022). In due course it will be documented in the written report sent to the referring medical practitioner, family doctor, family, and anyone else on the young person's treating team.

Our mind-body team finds it helpful to think of the assessment as a screening process, and the initial formulation as a working formulation — one that will be updated as more information becomes available. What this means is that as a clinician, you do not need to get all the historical information at the outset, and you do not need to get bogged down in details. You can always go back and get further information later if needed. It also means that you should be able to complete the assessment and formulation in the standard 60- to 90-minute time frame used by mental health clinicians.

It is important to note that antecedent stressors are no longer required for the diagnosis of functional seizures. This criterion was taken out of DSM-5 and ICD-11 because many adult patients did not report any antecedent psychological stressors. Through our work with young people, however, it is our clinical judgment (supported by our research experience) that presentations without any physical, psychological, educational, or relational stressors are very rare. As shall become evident throughout this chapter, functional seizures in young people are often triggered in the context of commonplace cumulative stressors: illness events, death of a grandparent, bullying at school, difficulties at school, friendship fallings-out, and so on.[1]

The Structure of the Initial Biopsychosocial Assessment with the Young Person and the Family

In our mind-body team, the structure of the biopsychosocial assessment involves six interconnected elements.

Construct the Genogram

Start with a three-generational genogram. The genogram is a basic tool in child and adolescent assessments and should include any deaths, any divorces, and where people live in relation to the young person. While drawing the genogram,

---

1 We have found the same pattern of findings across all our cohorts. For a recent study using the Early Life Stress Questionnaire (ELSQ) in children and adolescents with FND (and matched healthy controls), see Chung and colleagues (2022).

ask for a family medical history: begin with medical problems (including functional illnesses [see Figure 1.1]) and then ask about mental health problems — anxiety, depression, and so on — if they have not been touched upon already. The genogram will help with understanding what vulnerabilities the young person may have, but also help with beginning to build a picture of family stressors through illness, death, family cut-offs, and so on.

Elicit and Document the Young Person's Developmental Story

Complete the young person's developmental story. Start with the mother's pregnancy and move through each of the young person's developmental stages — or school years once you get to the school years — paying particular attention to nodal points: stress during the pregnancy, regulation in infancy (sleep, feeding, settling), separating as a toddler, starting preschool/childcare, starting school, reaching puberty, transitioning to high school.

The key goal of the family story is to understand the young person's experiences — both good and bad — during her development.[2] When were things going well? When did life challenges weave their way into the story? What levels of stress did the young person experience? When did the stress go up, and when did it go down? How high up did it go? How did the young person respond to this stress? How did her body respond? Whom did she talk to? Was she able to obtain support and help? What was the experience of other family members?

In order to tap into the emotional aspect of this story, it can be useful to ask about the 'family temperature' at different times (a rating up to 10) (see Figure 3.1: temperature tool) or to use a Likert scale where the young person can mark her level of subjective stress (see Figure 3.2). Sometimes the young person will tell you that she is fine, but the markings on the Likert scale will help you and the family appreciate her actual level of felt stress.

Probe for Physical, Psychological, and Relational Stressors

While listening to the family story, probe for stressors — physical, psychological, educational, and social and relational. Common physical stressors can include a viral illness, minor injury, vaccination, or medical procedure. We highlight physical stressors repeatedly throughout this manual because mental health clinicians — who are more likely to focus on psychological factors — need to ensure that they identify any physical stressors in the developmental story.

When exploring the young person's perspective, pay attention to, and ask about, the following: bullying or teasing, learning difficulties, demands for high

---

2 As noted in earlier chapters, because functional somatic symptoms occur more frequently in girls than in boys, we generally use the pronouns she and her to reflect this clinical reality.

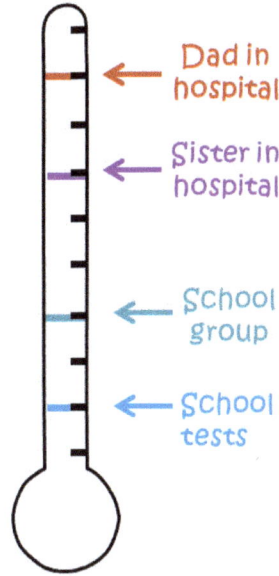

Figure 3.1 Family temperature tool. The temperature tool can be used during the assessment process to quantify the levels of family stress — 'family temperature' — at different times during the child's developmental story. © Kasia Kozlowska 2019

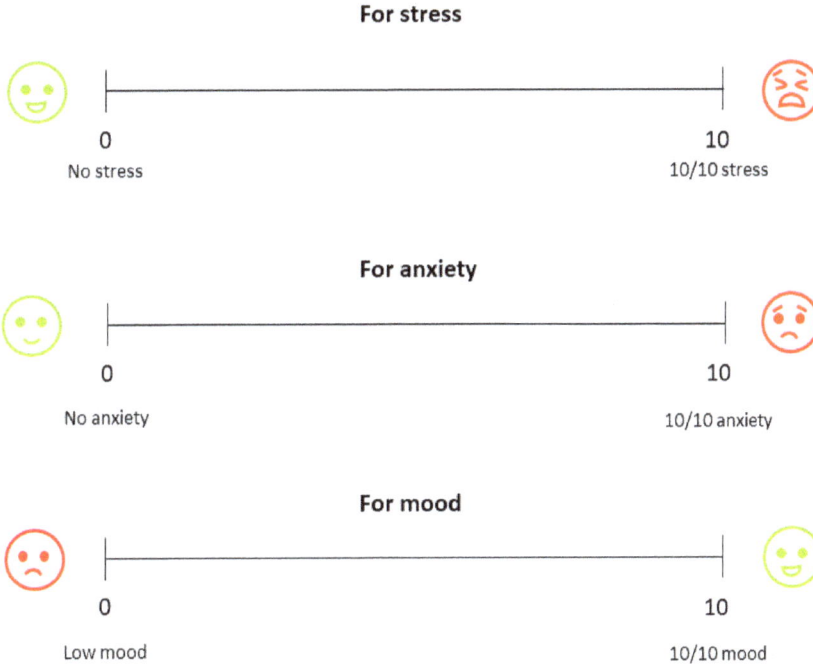

Figure 3.2 Likert scales for stress, anxiety, and depression. A simple Likert scale can be used to quantify the level of stress, anxiety, and depression felt by the child. It is particularly useful in identifying changes in levels of stress, anxiety, and depression over time (e.g., Year 1, Year 2, Year 3, and so on, of school). © Kasia Kozlowska 2022

academic achievement, fallings-out with friends (social rejection), tensions in sibling relationships, physical illness or injury, loss or trauma events, stress levels at school or home at different points in the story (e.g., using a simple Likert scale) (see Figure 3.2).

When exploring the family perspective, pay attention to, and ask about, the following: family illnesses, family deaths, parental job loss or change, parental separation, and levels of family stress at different points in the story (see Figures 3.1 and 3.2).

Because the young person's experiences are embodied, the stress-related aspect of the story will provide you with information about the challenges that activated her stress system, whether she was able to manage these challenges, and whether the challenges exceeded her ability to cope and were expressed as functional symptoms.

Integrate the Somatic Symptoms into the Story

Integrate a stress-symptom timeline into the family story; that is, identify the developmental time points at which the young person experienced stress-related somatic symptoms. For example, if the family is telling you about a difficult event in the family story — especially an event that the young person found to be stressful — ask how she responded and, in particular, whether she displayed any stress-related symptoms. Did the young person's sleep become disturbed? Did she experience any headaches or tummy pains? Did her eating patterns change? Did she feel sick in the mornings before school? Did she experience any stress-related gut symptoms (nausea, vomiting, or disruption of regular bowel function)? And so on.

Probing for these stress-related symptoms allows you to build a timeline of the young person's stress symptoms that runs alongside the family story. Very often you will find that the young person's functional somatic symptoms have a long history — and one interconnected with the history of the family.

Screen for Comorbid Anxiety, Depression, and Other Mental Health Disorders

All young people should be screened for anxiety and depression. This information may come out during the family story, or it may need to be explicitly asked about.

To screen for anxiety, you could ask the young person to rate her anxiety/worry on a Likert scale of 1 to 10, with follow-up questions if needed (see Figure 3.2). You can ask, for example, whether worries ever keep her up at night or distract her in class.

To screen for depression, you could ask the young person to rate her mood on a Likert scale of 1 to 10, with a risk assessment if indicated (see Figure 3.2).

It can also be helpful to ask about anxiety or mood at different points in the story — for example, Year 5, Year 6, and Year 7 at school — to obtain a sense of the young person's health and wellbeing over time. As noted above, sometimes the young person will tell you that she was 'fine' at some particular time, but the markings on the Likert scale will help you and the family recognise that she was struggling.

Identify Markers of Stress-System Dysregulation

Finally, the young person should be assessed for biological markers of stress-system dysregulation. Specifically, she should be asked about her appetite and eating patterns, sleep, frequency of exercise, and presence of common stress symptoms — disrupted sleep, tummy pains, nausea, thumping heart, headaches or other pain, fatigue, and so on.

The young person can also be assessed for *hyperventilation*. High respiratory rates are a good marker of hyperventilation, the consequence of activating the respiratory motor system alongside autonomic arousal. She can be asked to count her resting breathing rate in the assessment session (how many breaths does she take in one minute). For children over six years of age, respiratory rates >25 breaths per minute are in the ≥97.5th centile, and respiratory rates >30 breaths per minute in ≥99.9th centile — that is, outside of what is healthy and normal (Fleming et al., 2011; Wallis et al., 2005). The information about hyperventilation is important to elicit in young people presenting with functional seizures because our clinical research showed that about 50% of children and adolescents with functional seizures trigger their seizure events by hyperventilation: hyperventilation increases brain arousal and makes neural networks[3] more unstable (Kozlowska, Rampersad, et al., 2017).

Some clinicians will also assess *heart rate variability* using a biofeedback device. Heart rate variability is a proxy measure of restorative parasympathetic activity — the calming component of the autonomic nervous system. Heart rate variability is high when a young person is in a relaxed and calm state, and low when she is in a state of high arousal. If the young person is able to increase her heart rate variability with paced (slow) breathing, then she has good capacity to activate restorative processes to calm the autonomic nervous system. An inability to slow the breath or to increase heart rate variability suggests a state

---

3 Alternative terminology for neural networks — when talking to younger children — includes *brain networks*, *brain systems*, or just *the brain*

of overactivation that the young person finds difficult to settle. For a detailed discussion about the autonomic nervous system, see Chapter 6 of Kozlowska, Scher, and Helgeland (2020).

Building a Shared Formulation

One of the goals of the biopsychosocial assessment is to reach a shared biopsychosocial formulation with the young person and the family. When the biopsychosocial assessment is undertaken in the form of the collaborative storytelling process described above, the young person and family have multiple opportunities to recognise the link between challenging events in the young person's history and the body's reaction to those events. Many families experience an 'aha' moment when recurring patterns become clear to them. Other families struggle to make the links and find the process of building a shared formulation challenging but nevertheless, in the end, both helpful and necessary. This process — the building of the shared formulation — involves melding together the family story (= what the family knows) with what you, the clinician, bring to the encounter (= what you know). In a nutshell, the following points will need to be covered:

- Functional seizures occur when the young person's neural networks overactivate and become dysregulated in the context of high arousal — that is, when the brain-body stress system goes into overdrive, presenting as a functional seizure.

- You and the family can talk through the events that the family have described that may have switched on the young person's stress system earlier in development, thereby making her more sensitive to subsequent stress.

- You can talk through the biological markers indicating that the young person's stress system is switched on: dysregulated sleep, nightmares, disturbed appetite, history of headaches, history of tummy pains, fatigue, hyperventilation, panic attacks (a thumping heart and feeling sweaty), difficulties in increasing heart rate variability using biofeedback, and so on.

- The body has 'calming systems' that are meant to turn on after the stress systems are activated and help the stress systems 'switch off', allowing the body to calm down. For some people who have experienced a lot of stressors, the calming systems stop working well, and the stress systems do not switch off when they should.

- Treatment therefore includes interventions that help the young person become more skilled at reading her body state — for example, when the body stress systems are activating — and strategies to 'switch off' the stress systems and to strengthen the calming systems.

For the interested clinician, our mind-body team has written up detailed examples of the co-constructed biopsychosocial formulations in children and adolescents presenting with functional neurological disorder (FND). See the case study of Paula in Kozlowska, Scher, and Helgeland (2020) and our series of published case studies (Chandra et al., 2017; Chudleigh et al., 2013; Khachane et al., 2019; Kozlowska et al., 2016; Ratnamohan et al., 2018; Rajabalee et al., 2022).

Agreed Treatment Plan

Following the formulation, you can discuss the treatment plan with the family. Discussion of the following points can be helpful:

- The treatment plan is a 'mind-body' intervention designed to help the young person learn to regulate all levels of her body's stress system — that is, both body (including the brain) and mind.

- Treatment includes multiple components — including the biological, psychological, and social system levels (biopsychosocial) — and is most effective when the young person and family complete all the recommended components.

- Treatment components typically include the following: regulation of sleep and the circadian clock, exercise, individual psychology sessions, family work that supports the therapeutic process, and school attendance (if an inpatient, at the hospital's own school). When indicated, treatment may also include the use of medication.

- The family and clinician need to reach an agreement concerning the professionals who will make up the young person's treatment team — that is, which clinicians will provide which component of the treatment intervention.

Examples of Biopsychosocial Formulations for the Assessment Report

The formulation co-constructed with the family during the biopsychosocial assessment is documented in the assessment report. The report provides the family, the referring medical team (or neurologist or other medical practitioner), and the clinicians who make up the multidisciplinary treatment team with a shared understanding of the factors that contributed to the development of the functional seizures in the young person. Below are several examples of formulations co-constructed with the young person and the family and then formally documented via the assessment report.

Formulation Example 1: A Teenage Girl Presenting with Cumulative Stressors

Jane is a 15-year-old adolescent girl who was referred by Dr. A (paediatric neurologist) to the mind-body team for assessment and treatment of functional seizures. Functional seizures occur when brain stress systems become overactivated and interfere with motor-processing regions of the brain. Overactivation of brain stress systems can occur due to physical, psychological, or relational stressors. In Jane's case, overactivation of her brain stress systems appears to have been triggered by a viral infection (physical stressor) that activated her stress system in the context of cumulative psychological stressors: long-term, untreated anxiety; her being diagnosed with cancer (18 months ago); and reintegration into her local school following treatment for the cancer. Jane reported that she had experienced panic attacks throughout her life, often up to 3–4 times a week. Despite these challenges, Jane has numerous positive supports, including supportive parents and good friendships at school, and she has expressed a desire to engage in treatment for both her anxiety and functional seizures.

Formulation Example 2: A Teenage Girl Presenting with Functional Seizures and Epileptic Seizures

Kate is a 13-year-old girl who was referred by Dr. B (paediatric neurologist) to the mind-body team for assessment and treatment of recent-onset functional seizures, against a background of epilepsy and learning difficulties. Kate's *epileptic* seizures, diagnosed by the neurology team when Kate was three years old, present as absence seizures. Her *functional* seizures present as jerking movements in her arms and legs, sometimes accompanied by slurred speech. Kate's parents are confident that they are able to differentiate the functional seizures from the epileptic seizures.

Functional seizures are a form of neural network dysregulation. They are caused by overactivation of brain stress systems that are 'switched on' by stress and unable to 'switch off'. Functional seizures can be triggered by psychological stress (e.g., strong emotions like worry, distress, or not liking something) or physical stress (e.g., fatigue, pain, or hyperventilation). Female sex hormones also up-regulate the stress system and can increase the likelihood of functional seizures. The precipitating factors for Kate's functional seizures include onset of puberty (increase in female sex hormones) and the transition to high school (increased academic expectations). Moreover, the majority of Kate's functional seizures occur in the late afternoon and evening, when Kate is fatigued after the travails of the school day. She has fewer functional seizures on weekends.

The treatment for Kate's functional seizures is to increase the regulation in the brain and body and to help Kate to manage life challenges and difficult emotions. Treatment will involve helping Kate to manage distress, stress, and worry pertaining to school and the challenges of learning. It will also include her learning body-based regulation strategies that help her body calm down (e.g., through rocking, swinging, relaxation, stress balls, and slow-paced breathing).

Formulation Example 3: A Teenage Girl Presenting with Functional Neurological Disorder in the Context of Past Trauma

Xenia is a 14-year-old girl presenting with FND — leg weakness, nausea, dizziness, and functional seizures presenting as blackouts — following a netball injury. Xenia lives with her grandparents. Xenia also meets diagnostic criteria for posttraumatic stress disorder (PTSD; manifesting as nightmares and intrusive memories during the day) and postural orthostatic tachycardia syndrome (POTS; contributing to symptoms of dizziness and nausea on standing).

FND manifests when overactivated brain stress systems — overactivated in response to physical, psychological, or relational stress — interfere with and disrupt normal motor function, resulting in a myriad of functional neurological symptoms.

Xenia has experienced high levels of cumulative stress from three years of age. She, along with her siblings, has experienced the following: neglect (insufficient food coupled with a lack of appropriate adult supervision); repeated exposure to domestic violence (with fears that her siblings or mother would be irreparably injured by one of her mother's various male partners); and repeated house moves (making it difficult to maintain a friendship group and to keep up with academic demands at school). On moving in with her grandparents three years ago, Xenia suffered from trauma-related nightmares and hypervigilance to threat cues (symptoms of PTSD). These symptoms settled over a 12-month period, and Xenia was able to push the memories out of her mind. She was also able to make good progress at school.

Three weeks prior to Xenia's presentation with FND, she was reading the newspaper and saw a picture of one of the perpetrators, who had been arrested by the local police. The picture triggered a cascade of trauma-related memories. The memories emerged — night after night — in the form of nightmares. Three weeks later, a netball injury triggered various functional symptoms, including her functional seizures.

The treatment for Xenia's FND will involve a multidisciplinary approach: mind-body regulation strategies to calm the brain stress systems; physiotherapy to facilitate normal motor function; and high fluid intake, high salt intake, pressure socks, and slow-paced breathing to help regulate the POTS and her autonomic nervous system. Following the current intervention for FND, Xenia will need to engage in long-term psychotherapy — with a trauma-focused component — to process some of the trauma-related memories that currently function to activate her stress system on a daily basis (see Chapter 8 pertaining to illness-promoting psychological processes). Despite the challenges, ongoing efforts to maintain safety are also needed.

Formulation Example 4: A Teenage Boy Presenting with Functional Seizures and Neurodevelopmental Vulnerabilities

John is an 11-year-old boy with a diagnosis of FND presenting as functional seizures. John is a neurodevelopmentally vulnerable boy with pre-existing diagnoses of sensory processing disorder (including moderate speech delay), autism spectrum disorder (level 2), attention-deficit/hyperactivity disorder, and anxiety.

FND occurs when the brain stress systems become overactivated — and in the case of functional seizures, experience sudden increases in arousal and dysregulation — in the context of physical, psychological, or relational stressors. Some young people can trigger their functional seizures via anxious thoughts, catastrophising, anticipatory anxiety, or hyperventilation (a symptom of anxiety).

In John's case, he has a long-term history of anxiety (including separation anxiety) and a complex history of family stress. There are many family arguments and conflict at home, both between siblings and between the adults. John also reports finding school more challenging over time as the work increases in complexity and difficulty, which is further compounded by school absenteeism due to difficulties in managing his functional seizures.

In order to control his functional seizures, John needs to learn the skills of monitoring body arousal, including increases in anxiety. He also needs to learn self-regulation skills to reduce body arousal and anxiety — thereby averting the functional seizure. A regime of regular exercise (which is also regulating), good eating, and adequate sleep is also important.

The mind-body team needs to contact the school to work out a suitable learning plan and to ensure that John experiences his return to school as safe and predictable. The mind-body team also needs to refer John's parents to a family therapy service that can help them reduce family stress and manage conflict at home differently.

Potential Challenges That May Crop Up During the Initial Assessment

The Family Has Not Been Given a Clear Diagnosis

In the scenario where the family has not been given a clear diagnosis, you can direct the family back to the referring medical professional for diagnostic clarity. Common reasons for the failure to provide a clear diagnosis include the following: professional discomfort with providing a functional diagnosis because of perceived stigma or lack of skill (Kozlowska et al., 2021), pending medical investigations, and a mixed presentation that requires the functional elements to be carefully teased out. You need to support the family in their efforts to obtain or clarify the diagnosis because this is an important part of the assessment and treatment process. If necessary, you may need to help advocate for them to the medical professional who referred them to you. Do not take a position in which you argue with the family or try to convince them of the diagnosis. Making the diagnosis is not in your scope of practice. It is the responsibility of the neurologist or paediatrician.

The Family Does Not Accept the Diagnosis

If the family does not accept the diagnosis, you can direct the family back to the referring medical professional — or their family doctor — so that a second opinion can be organised. Again, it is helpful to support the family in their efforts to clarify the diagnosis because this is an essential part of the assessment and treatment process. It is very difficult for the young person and the family to commit to a therapeutic process if their perception of the problem differs from that of the clinician. Very rarely, a family is not able to accept the diagnosis despite multiple additional opinions, with the consequence that appropriate treatment cannot be provided to the young person. In that situation, the case may fall into the realm of child protection services (in Australia, available for children less than 14 years old).

The Pitfall of Trying to Get an Overly Comprehensive History or Perfect Formulation Before Starting Treatment with the Young Person

Clinicians working in some psychological services have a preference for a long assessment process that is undertaken over many sessions. Running such an assessment when the presenting symptom is functional seizures — where the young person and family are eager for the treatment to commence — runs the risk of losing engagement with the young person and family. We recommend doing a good-enough assessment in 60–90 minutes, to provide a working biopsychosocial formulation and to enable treatment to begin promptly. You can revise the working formulation as new information comes to light over the course of treatment.

The Pitfall of Trying to Uncover Hidden Trauma

The outdated aetiological model of functional seizures — based on Sigmund Freud's early work — held that they were caused by deep-seated, often unconscious traumas. Current research with children and adolescents does not support this model. Current research shows, instead, that in the majority of cases, functional seizures are triggered in the context of commonplace cumulative stressors (e.g., illness events, death of a grandparent, bullying at school, difficulties at school, and friendship fallings-out). Only a small percentage of young people report maltreatment or other major trauma (Chung et al., 2022). Unfortunately, some clinicians still follow an outdated model of functional seizures and will therefore try to uncover hidden trauma during their assessments. Moreover, the clinician may mistakenly believe that the young person is dissembling when she cannot disclose the trauma.[4] Such unproductive interactions generally lead families to become swiftly disengaged in the treatment process and reluctant to seek help from other clinicians working in psychological services.

The Family Are Not Willing or Not Able to Share Their Story

Sometimes the young person and the family are not forthcoming with their story. This makes it very difficult for the clinician and family to co-construct a biopsychosocial formulation. Some families or family members are not forthcoming because they do not wish to share information. The information may be pushed out of mind because it is too painful or embarrassing, or a closely guarded secret. Sometimes the negative experience in the medical system may make it difficult for the family — having been harmed by previous experiences — to trust the health professional(s) (Kozlowska et al., 2021). Sometimes information is not shared because the young person does not realise that anything is wrong. Nothing has changed in her experience of the family; from her perspective, the experience is normative. It may be many years — following exposure to other relationships and families — before the young person becomes aware of unhelpful dynamics that were previously masked or invisible.

If the family is still willing to work with you, you can still put together a working formulation and agree to a treatment plan. For example, you may say to the family:

---

4 See, for example, the story of Samantha in Chapter 2 of Kozlowska, Scher, and Helgeland (2020) or the case vignettes in Kozlowska and colleagues (2021).

> We know from Susan's increased breathing rate, poor sleep, and
> nausea that Susan's body is very up-regulated. But at the current
> time we don't have a full understanding of what might be
> activating her body. How about we start to work on mind-body
> strategies to help Susan begin the task of regulating her body . . .
> You never know; as we work together we might be able to figure
> out some of the things that have activated her body.

In subsequent sessions and conversations with the family, you can leave lots of
spaces and opportunities for the family to talk about their story if they choose
to do so. Some families will never disclose the story. For others it comes out in
dribs and drabs, or even years after treatment has been completed. From the
clinician's point of view, not knowing the family story can make treatment
more difficult, prolonged, and cumbersome. Despite these difficulties the
young person can still make significant clinical gains.

The Hostile Family

Some families are hostile and resentful of being referred to clinicians working
in psychological services. Often this can be because the patient has been
explicitly or implicitly told that functional seizures have a psychological cause
or that it is 'all in her head'. Alternatively, the family may have been told that
the young person is faking the functional seizures or that the young person is
being overly dramatic.[5] Even if these are not the explicit messages that a
medical professional has given to a family, the family may interpret any
references to 'psychological causes' as just indicated. An assessment using the
Stress-System Model can often defuse the hostility from these families and give
them a different understanding of functional seizures. You may need to spend
more time on psychoeducation in the initial assessment with these families, and
less time on the developmental history. It can also be helpful to state upfront
that when you use the term *stress*, you refer to all events — physical, psychological, educational, and social and relational — that the young person experiences
as stressful. In this light, a viral infection and a falling-out with a friend are both
experienced as stressful, and both function to activate the stress system.

Gathering Collateral Information

As with any good biopsychosocial assessment where the presenting patient is
a young person, it is important — with the family's consent — to gather
collateral information. At a minimum, you should speak with staff from the

---

5 For case examples see Kozlowska and colleagues (2021).

young person's school (looking ahead, this contact helps to establish the foundation for a school-based health care plan for managing the functional seizures, without which the young person will be unable to return to school [see Chapter 13]). You should also speak to any other mental health clinicians that the young person has recently had contact with. Likewise, for families who have a long-term family doctor, valuable information can be obtained from that source.

Chapter 4

Psychoeducation

The goals of psychoeducation are to explain to the family and young person what functional seizures are and to help them understand the rationale for the treatment program. In addition, it is important to provide the young person with information about terminology in order to avoid confusion, particularly if other health professionals have used different terms.

Before we move on, we should remind the clinician reader that we use the terms *stress system* (singular) and *stress systems* (plural) interchangeably. Sometimes we refer to the stress system as a whole (stress system) and sometimes to one or more subsystem components (stress systems) that make up the stress system (see Figure 1.3 on page 7).

What Are Functional Seizures?

In this section we list some of the key elements of functional seizures — elements that are often included in psychoeducation with the young person and her family.[1] We also provide you, the reader, with a simple explanation of functional seizures in Text Box 4.1. Appendix B is a fact sheet about functional seizures suitable for printing. Translations into some other languages are available online. See Appendix B for information on how to access these.

Text Box 4.1
A Simple Explanation of Functional Seizures

'We know that brain networks activate with stress. When your brain networks activate too much and for too long, normal brain function is disrupted, and a functional seizure can emerge.'

---

1 As noted in earlier chapters, because functional somatic symptoms occur more frequently in girls than in boys, we generally use the pronouns she and her to reflect this clinical reality.

Key psychoeducation information pertaining to functional seizures includes the following:

- Functional seizures reflect excessive activation and temporary dys-regulation of neural networks (or when using simpler language with younger children, brain networks, brain systems, or simply the brain).

- Functional seizures are triggered by stress — physical, psychological, or both.

- The brain is very sensitive to stress, both physical and psychological. When the stress system is activated — either by one big stressor or by lots of little stressors over time — the body (including the brain) can respond by manifesting stress-related symptoms, including functional seizures.

- When a young person experiences a functional seizure, she loses control of her body and may experience abnormal movements, loss of body tone, difficulty thinking clearly, and sometimes a loss of consciousness or a change in the level of consciousness.

- The physical stressors that can trigger a functional seizure are diverse (see Figure 4.1). Physical stressors are thought to trigger functional seizures because they activate the stress systems bottom-up via neurophysiological processes. In addition, the anticipation or experience of physical stressors may activate cognitive (mind-related) processes — negative thoughts and feelings in relation to the physical stressor — which, in turn, will activate the stress system top-down (see Chapter 8) (Gianaros & Wager, 2015). For example, the sensation of pain or the sight of blood during insertion of a cannula for a medical procedure may activate the stress system (especially the autonomic component) bottom-up, and the antici-patory fear may activate the stress system top-down.

- The psychological stressors that can trigger a functional seizure are also diverse (see Figure 4.1). Psychological stress — materialising in the form of negative thoughts and feelings — emerges when adverse events, challenges of daily living, or the build-up of such events overwhelms the young person's ability to cope. These cognitive (mind-related) processes function to activate the stress system top-down (see Chapter 8) (Gianaros & Wager, 2015). Psychological stress is person-specific. For example, end-of-year exams may be experienced as an interesting challenge by one child and as an over-whelming challenge and burden by another.

- Because many psychological stressors are associated with events and real-life challenges, they are sometimes also referred to as family stress, relational stress, school stress, academic stress, sport-related stress, and so on.

- Functional seizures are not dangerous: they do not cause any injury to the young person's brain.

- Young people with functional seizures have a very good prognosis if they engage in appropriate treatment. We expect young people who engage in and complete a treatment program to recover from their functional seizures. This is different from *adults* with functional seizures, who show lower rates of recovery.

- Functional seizures are a subtype of *functional neurological disorder* (FND) (see Figure 1.1 on page 2). Parents may be told that their child has 'FND presenting as functional seizures' or just that she has functional seizures — they are the same thing.

- It is common for functional seizures to change in the way they present; that is, their clinical presentation can change over time. This potential for variation is different from epileptic seizures, which more typically have a repeating (stereotyped) pattern of presentation.

Four additional explanations accompanying four different visual metaphors are provided later in this chapter (see the legends for each of the visual metaphors).

Common physical stressors	Common psychological stressors
• Pain • Fatigue • Dysregulated sleep or too little sleep • Hyperventilation (breathing too fast increases activation [arousal] of neural networks) • An illness event (e.g., a viral illness) • A minor injury (e.g., a fall or broken limb) • A medical procedure • Pushing the body too hard physically (e.g., for a sporting competition) • An accident	• Related to family: family conflict, divorce, parental mental illness, loss of a loved one through death or separation • Related to peer relationships: bullying, exclusion by friends, loss of a friend who has moved away • Related to school: starting a new school, academic stress • Related to the young person's mental health: anxiety, depression, and so on

Figure 4.1 Common stressors associated with functional seizures.

The Many Different Names Used for Functional Seizures

Because it has taken the medical profession so long to begin to understand the neurobiology of functional seizures, they have been given many different names (see Figure 4.2) at various times in the past. Many of the names — often still in use — reflect the then-current, but now outdated, medical beliefs about what was causing such seizures. This profusion of names can be confusing to the young person and her family, who can sometimes mistakenly think that she has been diagnosed with multiple different conditions instead of one condition with different names. In this context it is helpful to inform the family about some of the different names.

Although we use the term *functional seizures*, common alternatives used in contemporary medicine include *non-epileptic seizures* and *dissociative seizures*, and when talking to young children, *stress seizures*. There are ongoing debates about terminology and the best terms to use (Wardrope et al., 2021). It is possible that the terminology will continue to change over time.

How Are Functional Seizures Different from Epileptic Seizures?

Functional seizures are time-limited episodes of neural network dysregulation — loss of balance and synchrony — that occur in the context of high arousal. Arousal, in the brain and body, increases in response to the challenges of daily living — that is, in response to physical or psychological stress. In the normal course of events, arousal increases in response to the challenge — to activate the body and brain and prepare it for action — and then decreases (down-regulates) back to baseline. But young people with functional seizures activate their systems — including neural networks — into a state of overdrive and temporary dysregulation. Given this dysregulation, the treatment of functional seizures includes mind-body strategies that decrease arousal, facilitate regulation, and decrease energy use (see next section about energy regulation).

By contrast, epileptic seizures are caused by sudden, abnormal electrical discharges in the brain. Epileptic seizures are therefore treated with medication that helps dampen the electrical activity. Because a small subset of epileptic seizures are caused by epileptogenic lesions — areas of abnormal brain tissue from which abnormal electrical discharges originate — some young people are treated with neurosurgery, which removes the abnormal tissue. See Text Box 4.2 for the difference between epileptic and functional seizures. See also Chapter 2 for discussion pertaining to the medical process by which functional seizures are diagnosed and distinguished from epileptic seizures by the neurologist.

Term used	Meaning of term/origin of term
Functional seizures	*Functional* is used by many clinicians because it denotes that functional seizures are part of FND and other functional disorders (see Figure 1.1).
Non-epileptic seizures/non-epileptic events/non-epileptic spells	This denotes the information that the seizures are not epileptic. It is used in DSM-5.[a]
Dissociative (non-epileptic) seizures or dissociative convulsions (a synonym for seizure)	This denotes the information that the functional seizures are a form of dissociation (a state of changed brain function). This is used in ICD-11.[b]
Stress seizures	This denotes the idea that the seizures are caused by physical or psychological stress.
Functional neurological symptom (conversion) disorder with non-epileptic seizures	This denotes that functional seizures are classified under the broader umbrella of functional neurological symptom (conversion) disorder, previously called *conversion disorder*, in DSM-5.[c]
Dissociative neurological symptom disorder with non-epileptic seizures	This denotes that functional seizures are classified under the broader umbrella of dissociative neurological symptom disorder in ICD-11.[b]
Pseudoseizures	This denotes the idea that the seizures look like epileptic seizures but are not epileptic seizures.
Psychogenic seizures/psychogenic non-epileptic seizures/psychogenic non-epileptic events	This denotes the idea that the seizures are caused by a psychological process (but it does not account for seizures triggered by physical stressors such as pain, hyperventilation, or states of high arousal).
Non-epileptic attacks/non-epileptic attack disorder (NEAD)	This term was created in order avoid using the term *seizure* and thereby confusing functional seizures with epileptic seizures.
Conversion disorder with attacks or seizures	This term denoted that functional seizures were classified under the broader umbrella of conversion disorder (older term for FND) in previous versions of DSM.
Hysterical convulsions	This denotes the idea that the seizures were part of hysteria (the old name for FND), when it was believed — from the time of the ancient Greeks — to be manifest only in women and to be caused by a wandering womb (μστέρα [hystera] in Greek).

[a] DSM-5 = *Diagnostic and Statistical Manual of Mental Disorders*, 5th Edition (American Psychiatric Association, 2013).

[b] ICD-11 = *International Statistical Classification of Diseases and Related Health Problems*, 11th Revision) (World Health Organization, 2018).

[c] Finding the term *functional neurological symptom disorder* cumbersome, clinicians around the world use the shorter form *functional neurological disorder* (FND).

Figure 4.2 The different names used for functional seizures. © Kasia Kozlowska 2022

Text Box 4.2
The Difference Between Epileptic Seizures and Functional Seizures

Epileptic seizures are caused by electrical discharges in the brain. Epileptic seizures are treated with medications that suppress those discharges. Functional seizures are caused by a dysregulation in brain networks caused by a state of high arousal — overdrive — in the context of physical, psychological, or relational stress. Functional seizures are treated with mind-body regulation strategies that decrease arousal and enable brain networks to settle (calm down).

Visual Metaphors for Functional Seizures

It can be helpful to use metaphors as part of psychoeducation. Four metaphors are offered below. The first three (Figures 4.3–4.5) were developed by our mind-body team. The fourth (Figure 4.6) was developed by the Salford Royal NHS Foundation Trust (2021).

Understanding the Rationale for the Treatment Program

In Chapter 3 we discussed the biopsychosocial assessment and the co-construction of a shared formulation with the young person and the family. When this process goes well, the family have an understanding of the various experiences — physical, family related, school related, friendship related — that the young person has struggled to manage and of how these experiences have functioned to activate the young person's stress systems, including the brain stress systems.

With the psychoeducation intervention (discussed in this chapter), the young person and family now also understand that activation of the brain stress systems can lead to an overactivation of brain networks — into a state of overdrive — causing temporary dysregulation that presents as functional seizures.

At this point in the process, it is important for the clinician to highlight that the treatment of functional seizures involves interventions — on a variety of system levels (body level, cognitive level, academic level, friendship level, or family level) — that help the young person increase her capacity to regulate her body and to manage stress and the challenges of daily living. And because the clinician has identified predisposing, precipitating, and perpetuating factors in the formulation, the clinician can use these to provide a rationale for treatment. Some examples that may be relevant to some — but not all young people — are:

- Because the young person has signs of increased arousal and motor activation — for example, high breathing rate — bottom-up regulation strategies targeting the body are likely to be helpful.

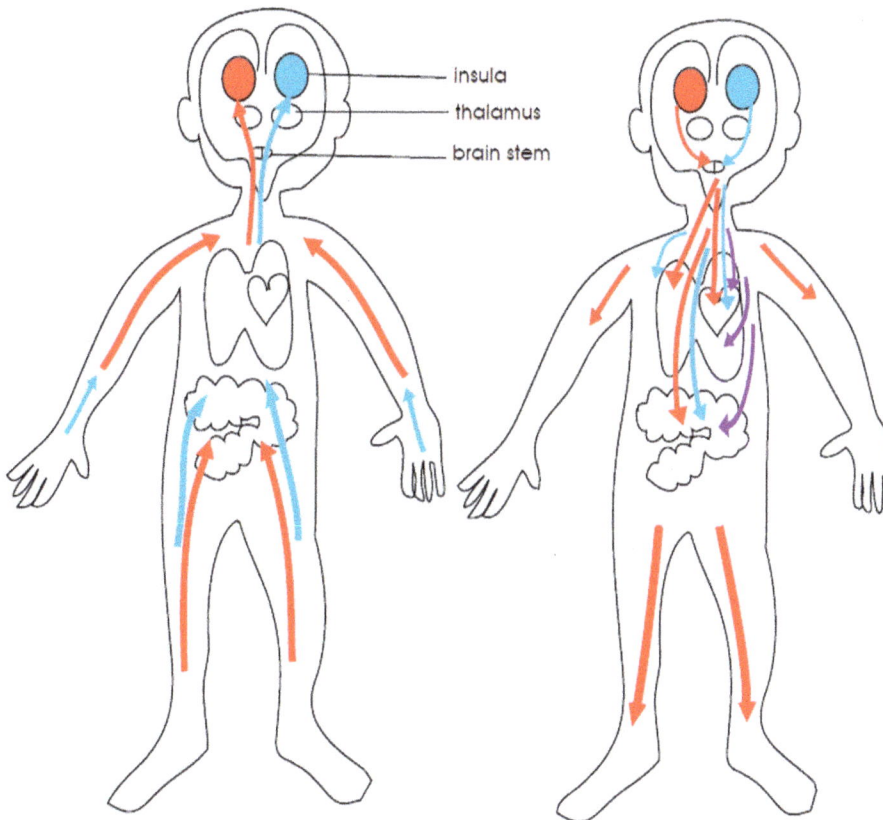

insula
thalamus
brain stem

Figure 4.3 Autonomic nervous system metaphor for functional seizures. In this simplified representation of the stress system in the body and brain, the red colour represents the sympathetic nervous system, the purple colour the defensive parasympathetic system, and the blue colour the restorative parasympathetic system. The red and purple colours indicate the part of the stress system that activates the body and brain in response to danger and stress (danger system). The blue colour indicates the part of the stress system that calms the body and brain. Functional seizures occur when the red system activates too much in the body and brain, and disrupts brain function. Treatment includes interventions that bring the blue system online. For a detailed description of the autonomic system and its components, see Chapter 6 in Kozlowska, Scher, & Helgeland (2020). © Kasia Kozlowska 2013

- Because the treatment of functional seizures includes implementation of strategies to avert the seizures, work on reading changes in body state is part of the treatment.

- Because the young person is deconditioned — has not done any exercise in quite a while — a physiotherapy intervention involving a regular exercise program is indicated. Regular pleasurable exercise helps regulate the stress system (see these physiotherapy-specific articles for more about physiotherapy in FND: Gray and colleagues [2020], Scheffer and colleagues [2020], and Kim and colleagues [2021]).

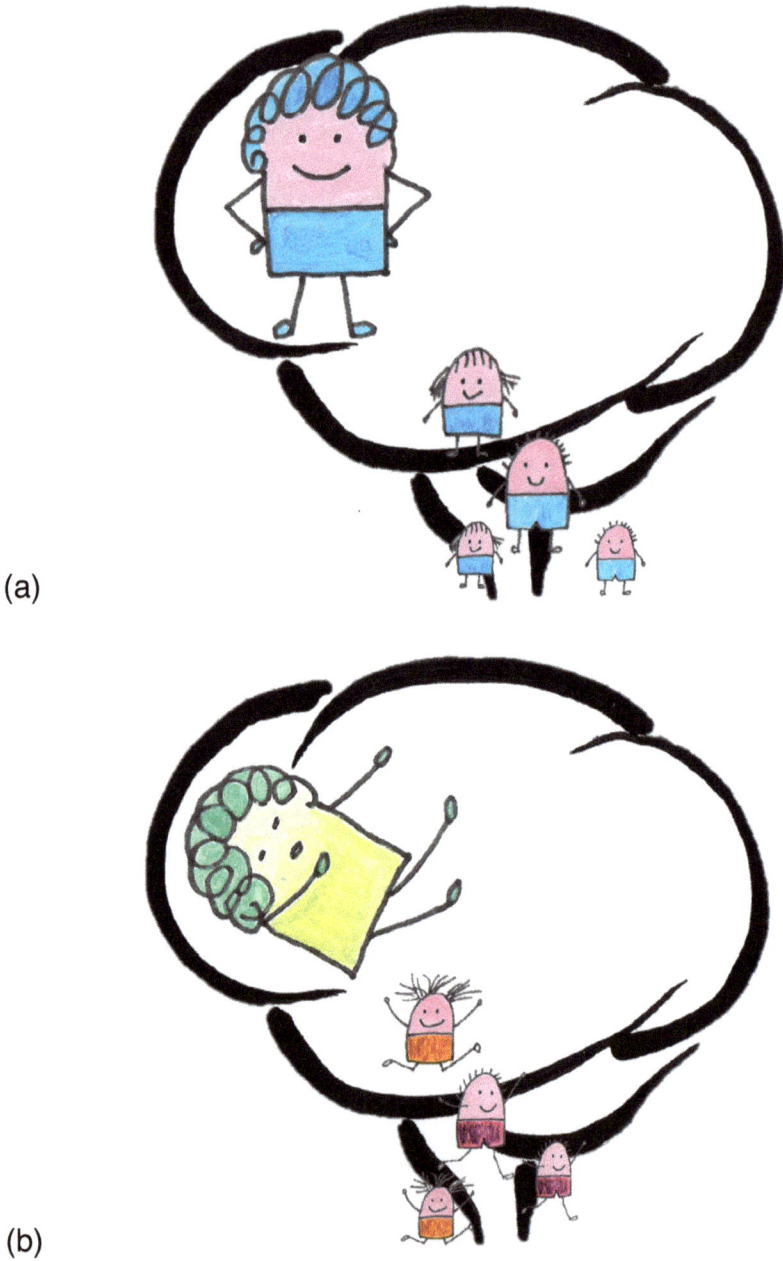

Figure 4.4 Children-going-wild metaphor for functional seizures. Visual representation of the hypothesised mechanism underpinning functional seizures. (a) The mother figure represents the prefrontal cortex, the control area of the brain. The child figures represent motor programs in the basal ganglia, midbrain, and brain stem. When all is well, the mother (prefrontal cortex) maintains control over the children (the motor programs), and she maintains regulation between brain networks. (b) In functional seizures, the mother (prefrontal cortex) goes offline in the context of stress-related changes. Regulation in the brain networks is lost, and the children (the motor programs) activate and present as functional seizures. © Kasia Kozlowska 2017

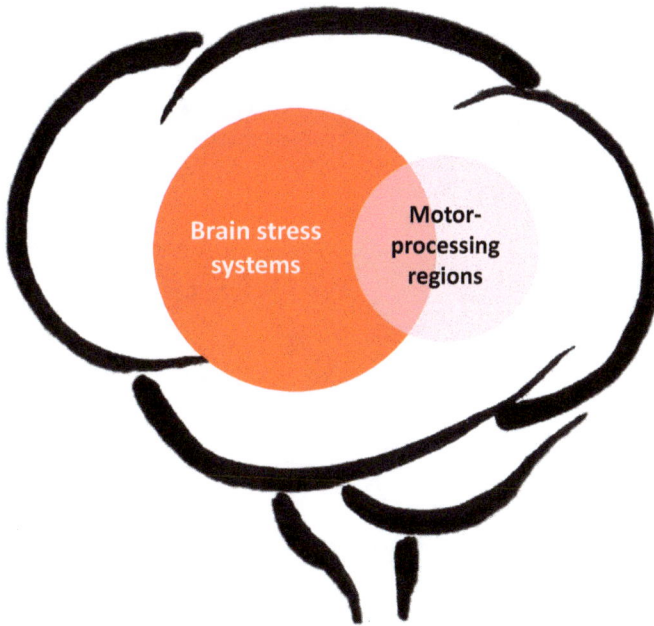

Figure 4.5 Brain stress systems metaphor for functional seizures. An alternative visual representation of the hypothesised mechanism underpinning functional seizures (based on emerging neuroscience research). The red ball represents the brain stress systems — the parts of the brain that activate with stress. When the red ball becomes too big and too strong, it can disrupt motor function (depicted by the pink ball). The red ball is activated by a broad range of physical (illness, injury, or medical procedure) or psychological stressors. The therapeutic intervention involves mind-body strategies that help the stress system settle down — the red ball to get smaller — so that the young person's functional seizures are no longer triggered. © Kasia Kozlowska 2017

- Because the young person ruminates and catastrophises — and these cognitive processes function to switch on the stress system — a cognitive intervention (e.g., cognitive-behavioural therapy [CBT]) is likely to be helpful. CBT interventions utilise top-down regulation strategies that target thoughts, feelings, and behaviours.

- Because the young person is struggling at school, a cognitive assessment is likely to clarify whether the young person has undiagnosed learning difficulties that may be contributing to her experience of the classroom as a source of stress.

- Because the young person is distressed when the family fights, a family intervention is likely to help family members manage conflict in a more productive way.

The Pressure Cooker Model

Pressure release valve 'closed' (preventing the release of stress)

For example: Always 'putting other people first'
No one to talk to about upsetting events
'Bottling up' feelings
Too busy to rest properly

Emotional stress released through mind-body link (e.g., functional seizures)

Emotional and physical stress building up in body

Stressful life events or ongoing difficulties

| Past stressful or traumatic situations | Current stressful situations | Mental health problems (e.g., low mood, anxiety) | Physical illness (e.g., pain, fatigue, poor health) |

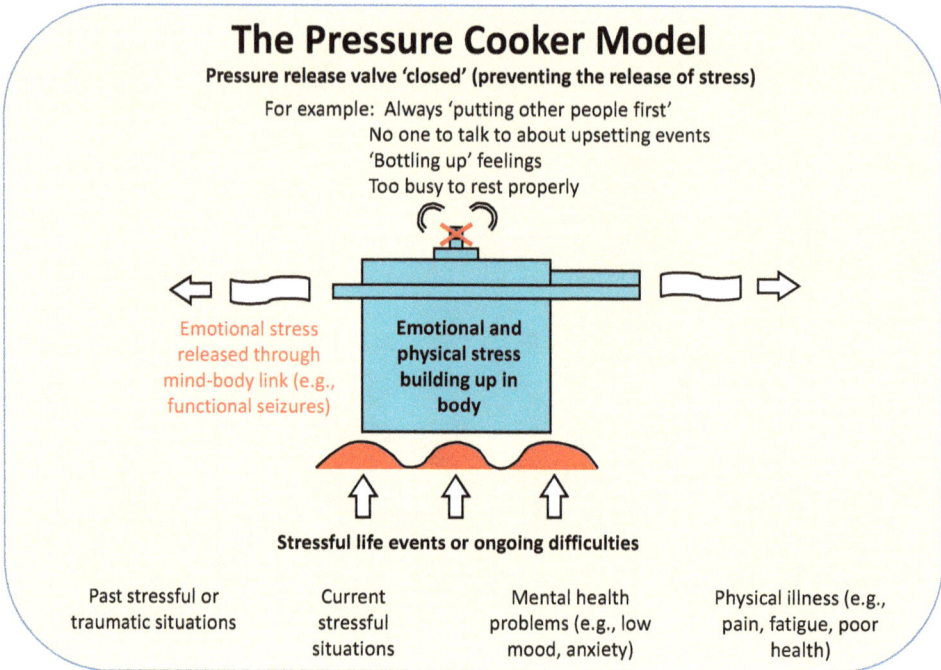

Figure 4.6 Pressure cooker metaphor for functional seizures. Functional seizures as a form of pressure cooker valve — a regulator of tension and arousal. Emotional and physical stress builds up in the body and brain. The functional seizures are protective. Their function is to avoid implosion. The pressure cooker lets off steam — in the form of functional seizures — to regulate arousal, enabling the overactivated brain to reset itself back to a regulated state. The young person must learn strategies to help the brain and body regulate and to better manage stress — and the challenges of daily living — that fuel the fire under the pressure cooker. This pressure cooker model is reproduced with permission from of Salford Royal NHS Foundation Trust.

Occasionally, the predisposing or precipitating factors may not be clear. In that scenario, it is helpful to be explicit that you and the young person may never find out exactly what triggered her functional seizures. Fortunately, however, it is now well known that the best treatment is to learn mind-body regulation strategies. These strategies help the overactive stress system regulate and to calm down.

Overview of Mind-Body Treatment Program

Here we provide some information tips directed to the young person that can be useful when discussing the treatment program with her, over and above the rationale for treatment:

- This treatment program will involve trying a range of different mind-body strategies to see which ones you like and which ones work for you. Most people find 2–3 strategies that they find helpful, and some people find even more.

- The treatment program involves practicing your strategies every day.

- Some parts of the program will be hard work (e.g., some people find going back to school hard or doing exercise hard); your family and your treating team will be there to help you with the hard bits.

- One of the first steps in the treatment program will be to learn to read your body's stress system. This will help you learn to identify your warning signs of a functional seizure and to practise using strategies to help your body calm down before having a functional seizure.

- The goal of this treatment program is to return to normal functioning and to do normal activities — to enable you to go to school, to go out with friends, and to be active.

Chapter 5

Re-establishing and Maintaining the Rhythms of Daily Living

Given that functional seizures reflect a temporary state of overdrive and dysregulation within neural (brain) networks,[1] a key intervention is to help the young person to draw on the body's own restorative and healing processes that are embedded in the daily rhythms of a healthy life. When activated on a daily basis, these restorative processes help down-regulate the stress system (and all its components). They help to calm it and keep it in check (see Figure 1.3). The rhythms of daily living include all of the following: a healthy sleep-wake cycle; healthy eating; regular, pleasurable exercise; and a daily routine that provides a rhythm to the day. It is important to inquire about each of these elements because, in a substantial proportion of young people with functional seizures, the elements are out of synchrony, have been put on hold, or reflect an ongoing problem area. Re-establishing these rhythms — creating repeating patterns (regulation) across the circadian cycle — is a necessary first step in the treatment process if the intervention for functional seizures is to succeed.

Regulating Sleep

One of the first steps in helping to regulate the young person's stress system — given the state of overdrive (arousal) in the brain and body — is to regulate sleep. A healthy sleep-wake cycle maintains circadian clocks in all tissues of the body, enables nocturnal restorative processes to be activated regularly, and ensures that the stress system (and all its components) is routinely 'switched off' during sleep (Chrousos et al., 2016; Kozlowska, Scher, & Helgeland, 2020) (see Figure 1.3). As a clinician, you can ask about difficulties falling asleep, waking in the night, difficulty returning to sleep, nightmares, difficulty waking in the

---

1 Alternative language for neural networks — when talking to younger children — includes *brain networks*, *brain systems*, or just *the brain*.

morning, sleeping during the day, sleep that is not restorative (i.e., you wake up and still feel tired), and excessive tiredness or fatigue.

Explain to the young person and her family[2] that, during sleep, the body activates its many restorative processes. Each night the stress systems are 'switched off'; the body's calming systems are 'switched on'; and the brain undergoes a 'sleep clean' where products of metabolism are flushed out and synapses are reset. These restorative processes rejuvenate the brain and body in preparation for the next day. If the young person is not sleeping properly, then her brain and body miss out on this process, and her stress systems and neural networks will be vulnerable to states of dysregulation, including functional seizures. Good sleep also increases the young person's capacity to learn mind-body regulation strategies, to have the energy and motivation to exercise, and to make healthy eating choices (Duraccio et al., 2022).

The young person and her family need to learn about sleep hygiene strategies (see Text Box 5.1). Since one important component of maintaining a regular circadian rhythm is exposure to sunshine in the morning, this should be included in the young person's sleep hygiene plan. Help the young person and family implement a sleep routine with a regular bedtime and a regular wake-up time.

A proportion of young people may have an inverted circadian rhythm: they sleep during the day and are awake at night (Chung et al., 2022). For these young people, the sleep routine may need to be reset so that it aligns with the day-night cycle. One way to reset the circadian clock is to go to sleep two hours later each day until the correct bedtime is reached. Another way to reset the circadian clock is for the young person to stay up all night and all of the subsequent day — to maximise sleep debt — and then to go to sleep at the correct bedtime.

If the young person's sleep is very dysregulated or does not seem to be responding to the suggested sleep hygiene strategies, she may need a medical review to consider medications to help with her sleep (see Chapter 15 about adjunctive use of medications).

For more information about the restorative functions of sleep, see Chapter 5 of Kozlowska, Scher, and Helgeland (2020). For further information about sleep hygiene measures, see handout from the Centre for Clinical Interventions (n.d.), Western Australia.

---

2 As noted in earlier chapters, because functional somatic symptoms occur more frequently in girls than in boys, we generally use the pronouns she and her to reflect this clinical reality.

Text Box 5.1
Basic Principles of Sleep Hygiene

- Go to bed and wake up at about the same time each night (including weekends).
- Have a regular ritual before bed to tell your body it is time to go to sleep.
- A warm bath or shower 1–2 hours before bedtime can help with falling asleep.
- Keep your bedroom dark, quiet, and cool.
- Avoid caffeine (in chocolate, tea, coffee, and some soft drinks) for 4–6 hours before bedtime.
- Limit naps to 20 minutes during the day.
- Don't have screen time 30–60 minutes before bed.
- Don't use screens in the bed.
- Don't lie in bed trying to fall asleep. If you aren't asleep in 20 minutes, do something different (e.g., read a book, listen to quiet music) and then try to go to sleep again.
- Go out in the sun first thing in the morning.

Regulating Eating

Healthy eating maintains a healthy microbiota-gut-brain axis and has far-reaching implications for physical and mental health (Pesheva, 2021). Some young people who have functional seizures also have dysregulated eating habits. For example, they may skip meals, have reduced appetite, or eat mainly unhealthy, processed foods. Assess for healthy eating by thoroughly exploring the young person's eating habits. Explain to her and the family that it is important to eat regularly in order to maintain healthy body rhythms, the energy resources needed for regular exercise, and the energy resources needed to learn and practise regulation strategies.

If you work in a medical setting, obtaining a routine weight and height allows you to calculate a body mass index and weight percentile — which informs you whether the young person is within or moving away from a normal, healthy range.

Discuss the importance of eating regular meals, even if these meals are small. Discuss the importance of eating at regular times. Eating regular meals at regular times gives the body the message that it is safe and being cared for (receiving regular sustenance). Regular eating also contributes to the daily routine — repeating patterns across the circadian cycle — that supports body regulation. Introduce the concept of the gut biome. While this research is in the early stages, the available evidence suggests that a healthy gut biome helps to regulate both the stress system and neural networks. Talk about maintaining a healthy gut biome — by eating enough fruit and vegetables, whole grains, and yoghurt. Tell the young person and family that the organisms that make up the gut biome also have a circadian rhythm (Li et al., 2018). They function best if they are fed regularly during the day and if they can rest and rejuvenate during the night. If these organisms are dysregulated because of unhealthy eating, then the brain and body will also be more vulnerable to dysregulation. If the young person is unable to eat regularly, options include drinking smoothies or even a meal supplement (e.g., Sustagen or Ensure) at mealtimes instead of a meal.

Regulating Activity/Exercise

Regular, pleasurable exercise helps to regulate the stress system. Each time we exercise, we activate the autonomic nervous system — alongside other systems — and then, when we are finished exercising, the autonomic nervous system down-regulates back to what is the current baseline for each person. In this way, regular exercise is, in and of itself, a regulation strategy. Regular exercise also maintains health in many other ways. It helps to maintain body conditioning; it activates the antioxidant system; and it activates other anti-inflammatory processes that promote neuroprotection (thereby down-regulating the inflammatory-immune component of the stress system) (Scheffer & Latini, 2020) (see Figure 1.3).

Young people who do not exercise become physically deconditioned, and their stress systems — and in particular, the autonomic nervous system component — become dysregulated. Many people with functional seizures have put all exercise 'on hold', often because they are afraid of inducing another functional seizure. Likewise, it is common for their parents to forbid exercise for fear of injury because of a functional seizure.

In a small handful of young people, exercise may potentially trigger functional seizures — either during the exercise itself or afterward (in the latter case because their stress systems, once activated by the exercise, fail to down-regulate).

Our team always recommends that the young person engage in regular daily exercise. The nature of this exercise will depend on how unwell and physically deconditioned the young person is. If the young person is very deconditioned, our team generally recommends starting with a small amount of regular exercise or activity (e.g., walking down the street) and slowly building up to the point of doing 30–60 minutes of exercise three to five times a week. Some young people may be so deconditioned — or so prone to functional seizures — that their exercise programs will begin with floor exercises only, thereby eliminating the risk of a fall. If the young person is exercising, just what exactly they do is secondary; the exercise can include anything from playing with a pet, to bushwalking, to trampoline jumping, to swinging on swings at the local park. Ideally, it should be an activity that the young person enjoys and finds pleasurable.

If the young person is very deconditioned or disabled due to functional seizures, she may need assistance from a physiotherapist or exercise physician in implementing an exercise program (Gray et al., 2020; Kim et al., 2021).

Putting Together a Timetable to Give a Rhythm to the Day

After reviewing the above three components — the regulation of sleep, eating, and exercise/activity — the therapist, family, and young person should develop a rudimentary daily timetable. The timetable can be adjusted day by day, week by week, or sometimes even month by month, and it should include sleep times, mealtimes, and exercise times. The timetable must be realistic for the young person to follow. If the timetable is too ambitious or not specific enough, it will not be containing — it will increase the child's anxiety, stress-system activation, and use of avoidance behaviours.

Over the course of treatment, the timetable will be enhanced and expanded into a daily therapeutic program that the young person follows. This first timetable becomes the basis for everything that follows. The timetable is the product of a collaborative process between the young person and therapist, and it is changed and supplemented over the course of treatment, evolving to address the changing capacities and challenges of each young person. An example timetable is included on the next page as Figure 5.1.

7.00 am to 7.30 am	Wake up
7.30 am to 8.00 am	Breakfast, get dressed, get ready for the day
8.00 am to 9.00 am	Leave for school
9.00 am to 3.00 pm	School (Eat morning tea and lunch)
3.00 pm to 4.00 pm	Travel home from school
4.00 pm to 4.30 pm	Afternoon tea
4.30 pm to 5.00 pm	Half an hour of exercise with mum (for example, walk the dog, jump on trampoline, or go for a swim)
5.00 pm to 6.00 pm	Homework (Monday, Tuesday, Wednesday) Gymnastics (Thursday) Youth Group (Friday)
6.00 pm to 7.30 pm	Free time
7.30 pm to 8.00 pm	Dinner
8.00 pm to 8.30 pm	Free time
8.30 pm to 9.30 pm	Start bedtime routine: Move phone out of room and log off any devices Have a cup of herbal tea Have a warm shower Read in bed
9:30 pm	Lights out and sleep

Figure 5.1 Example of an early daily timetable that supports the re-establishment of daily rhythms.

Chapter 6

The Five-Step Plan for
Managing Functional Seizures

Functional seizures are disruptive to the young person's life, and they cause a great deal of distress both for the young person and the family. Learning the skills to gain control over the functional seizures — and to be able to avert them — is the primary goal of the treatment intervention. The skills needed for a successful outcome are usually learnt in a stepwise manner.

Our mind-body team has operationalised these steps into a Five-Step Plan for Managing Functional Seizures (henceforth, the Five-Step Plan). Each step represents a piece of a complex therapeutic process whereby the young person — in collaboration with the therapist — develops a new skill set. Some young people progress through the five steps apace, over a period of weeks, and other young people will find the skills more difficult to learn and will take longer. A small subset of young people — those who present in a state of extreme arousal — may benefit from a concurrent pharmacotherapeutic intervention to help decrease their levels of arousal (see Chapter 15) during the time that they are engaged in mastering the skills of the Five-Step Plan.

The five steps of the plan (see below) are usually implemented sequentially. On occasion, however, the young person will struggle to master step 1, in which case the therapist needs to work on the skills pertaining to all five steps in parallel until the young person is able to consolidate the learning of the skill-building process. Visual representations of the Five-Step Plan are available in Appendix C (for the young person) and Appendix D (for the young person and parent [or other adult]). Both are suitable for printing, and translations of Appendixes C and D into some other languages are available online from the publisher.

Step 1 of the Five-Step Plan: Identifying the Warning Signs of a Functional Seizure

Identifying the warning signs of a functional seizure is the first step in the Five-Step Plan. Because many young people find this step challenging — and the therapeutic process that makes up this step is complex — we discuss it in detail. The key therapeutic ingredient of step 1 is the skill set of bottom-up mindfulness, which involves noticing and tracking the felt sense of the body, whether pleasant or unpleasant, with a curious, open stance (see Chapter 7 for more detail). The various ways of learning this skill are outlined below.

Psychoeducation

You, the clinician, may need to repeat some of the material that you covered previously in the psychoeducation process with the young person and the family. Remind the young person and her family[1] that functional seizures are not dangerous: they do not cause any injury to the young person's brain. Neural (brain) networks become overactivated, dysregulate in a temporary manner, and then reset themselves so that the young person can return to normal function.

The first step of the Five-Step Plan is to communicate to the young person how important it is to listen to her body and learn to identify the warning signs that a functional seizure may be about to occur. Because functional seizures occur in the context of brain and body arousal (activation), most young people are able, with time, to identify the signs and symptoms of increasing activation — what we call the *warning signs*. In other words, over time, the young person will become increasingly adept at noticing that her body is beginning to activate and to track the symptoms and signs associated with this activation. Once she can read her particular warning signs, the young person will need to start practising her mind-body strategies to try to settle her body and prevent the functional seizure from happening (see Chapters 7, 9, and 10).

Explain that learning to read the warning signs and using mind-body strategies to prevent the functional seizures will take time and practice. For this very reason, the young person will need to practise the skills she learns — listening to her body and implementing her mind-body strategies — on a daily basis during the treatment intervention.

Using a Body Map

Complete a body map with the young person (see Figure 6.1). Have the young person draw on the body map what happens in her body *immediately before* a

---

1 As noted in earlier chapters, because functional somatic symptoms occur more frequently in girls than in boys, we generally use the pronouns she and her to reflect this clinical reality.

functional seizure. Using a different colour, have her draw on the body map what happens in her body *during* a functional seizure. Then, using a third colour, have her draw on the body map what happens in her body *after* a functional seizure. Alternatively, you can represent this information of three different body maps. A blank body map (for filling in) is provided in Appendix E.

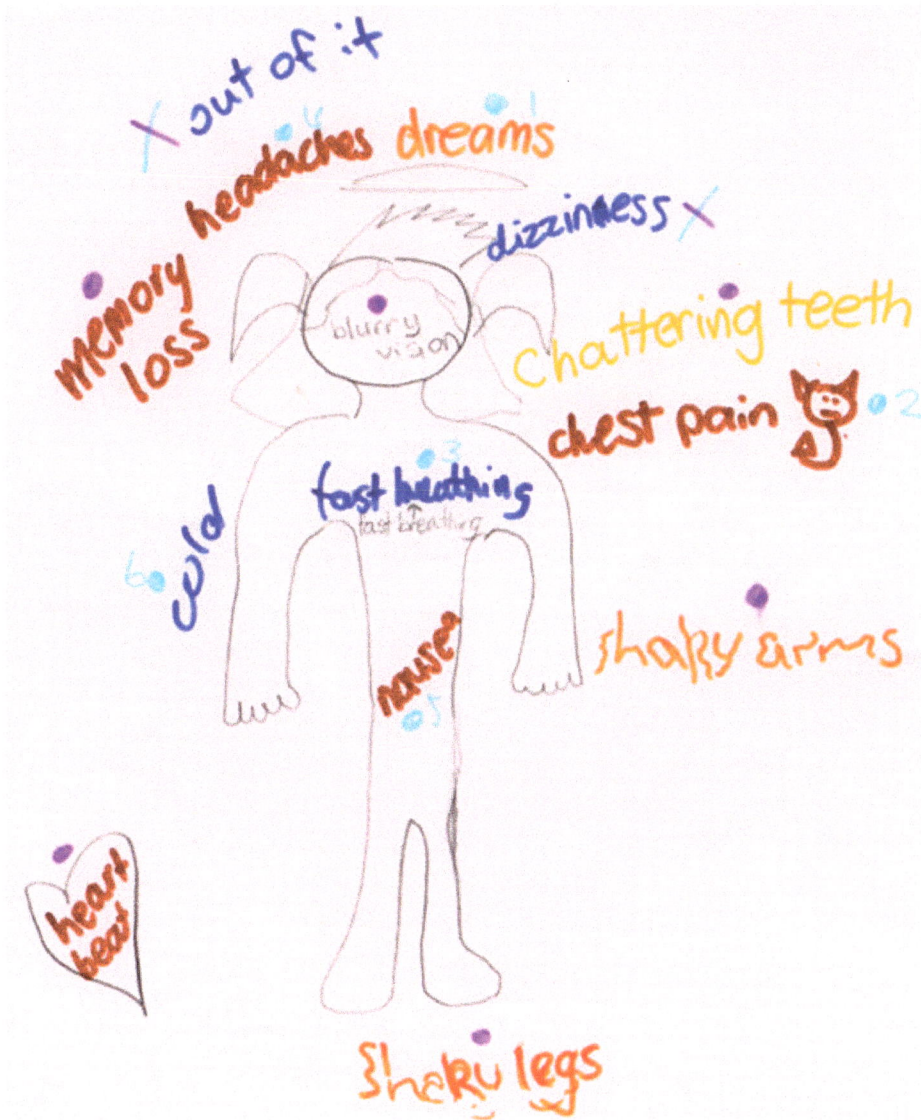

Figure 6.1 Body map representation of functional symptoms. This body map depicts all the functional symptoms experienced by a 12-year-old girl. © Kasia Kozlowska 2010

Do not be surprised if the young person struggles with this activity and cannot identify any warning signs. Explain that this is a work in progress and that the young person will keep adding information to the body map during the course of treatment. Make the positive prediction that you expect the young person to notice more warning signs over the course of treatment as the young person begins to take notice of what her body is doing. Keep the body map available in subsequent sessions so that when the young person notices any new bodily sensations, they can be added to the body map. Be sure to communicate your praise and encouragement for her increased body awareness.

For the young person who is very disconnected from her body, the daily practice of the body scan exercise (see Chapter 7) — with regular practice included into her daily timetable (see Chapter 5) — can help increase awareness of the felt sense of the body (body sensations), including the warning signs of a functional seizure.

Using Sequencing

Talk to the young person about the last time she had a functional seizure. Work backward from the functional seizure to identify warning signs. Use probing questions to explore what she was doing, thinking, and feeling, and what was happening in her body. Ask the young person to utilise any subsequent functional seizures as a learning exercise and to focus her attention on what happens in her body prior to and during subsequent functional seizure events. And be sure to add any newly identified details to the sequence of warning signs.

Here we note that the language used to describe the sequencing exercise varies within different schools of psychotherapy. Family therapists use the terms *sequencing* and *sequencing/tracking technique* (Lappin, 1988; Minuchin, 1974). Therapists working from the ethological tradition (Levine, 2010) and body-work traditions — including Eastern traditions — use the terms *tracking body sensations* and (bottom-up) *mindfulness* (Kain & Terrell, 2018; Levine, 2010; Ogden & Fisher, 2015). Therapists trained in Dialectical Behaviour Therapy (DBT) use the term *chain analysis* (Linehan, 2018; Rizvi, 2019).

Vignette: Evie

Evie, a 15-year-old girl, presented with functional seizures precipitated by chest pain (precordial catch syndrome) (Gumbiner, 2003; University of Wisconsin–Stevens Point Student Health Service, 2005). She reported that the chest pain came out of nowhere and that she could not identify any of the warning signs of her functional seizures. Evie said that when the chest pain occurred, she could do nothing to stop a functional seizure. Working backward from the time that Evie experienced the chest pain, the clinician and Evie worked together to ascertain the sequence of events that led up to it (see Figures 6.2 and 6.3). The sequence was drawn out on a large sheet of paper. Once Evie had identified some of the warning signs that her body experienced in the lead-up to the chest pain and functional seizure, she was able to practise noticing and labelling the body sensations. At this point Evie's therapist started to teach her neurophysiological regulation strategies to calm her body and avert some of the functional seizures.

In subsequent individual therapy sessions, Evie was also able to identify the thoughts that were part of the sequence (see Figure 6.4). Interestingly, early on during the sequence, Evie frequently thought, 'This isn't normal. I'm just going to ignore it. I don't want this to happen now.' This response enabled Evie to block out and to ignore her body's warning signs, which was why she had struggled so much to identify them to begin with. Evie and her therapist also determined that at other times, when the sensations became overwhelming and too strong to be ignored, Evie catastrophised her body's warning signs.

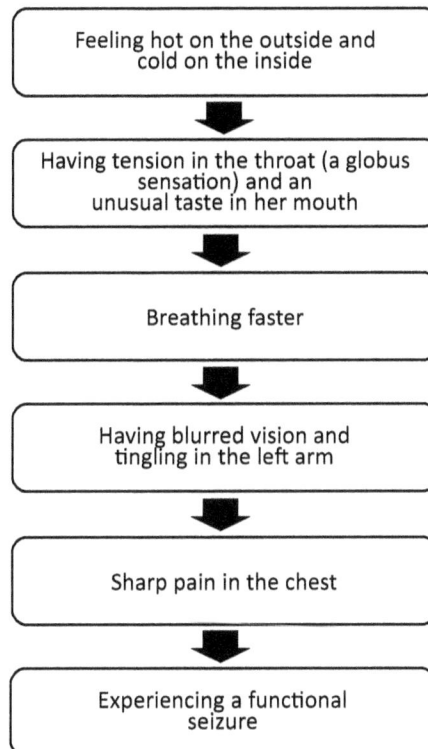

Figure 6.2 Evie's flowchart of warning signs. This flowchart documents the sequencing exercise done by Evie and her therapist. The flowchart shows the sequence of events — in terms of changes in body state (warning signs) — that preceded Evie's functional seizures. © Kasia Kozlowska and Blanche Savage 2022

Evie's somatic narrative	Clinician's interpretation
Feeling hot on the outside and cold on the inside	Sympathetic activation
Having tension in the throat (a globus sensation) and an unusual taste in her mouth	Increased tension in muscles of throat and sympathetic activation (dry mouth)
Breathing faster	Hyperventilation causing increased cortical arousal and activation of neural networks
Having blurred vision and tingling in the left arm	Peripheral symptoms of hyperventilation secondary to decreased cerebral blood flow (blurred vision) and hyperactivity of sensory nerves (tingling)
Sharp pain in the chest	Precordial catch pain— probably reflecting increased activation of muscles and fascia
Experiencing a functional seizure	Temporary dysregulation of neural networks

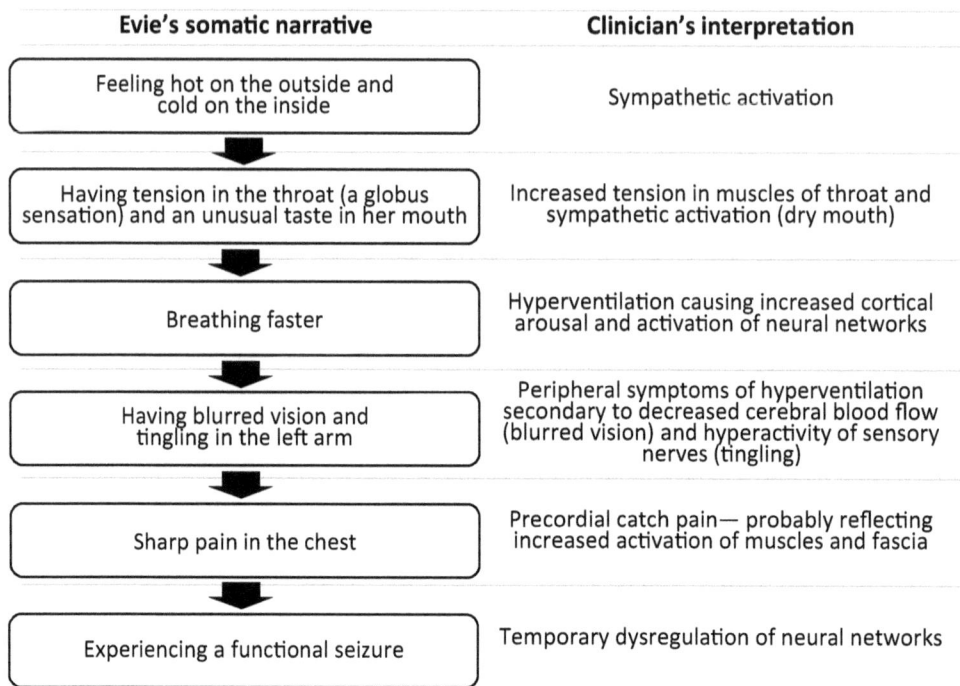

Figure 6.3 Evie's flowchart of warning signs with the clinician's neurophysiological inter-pretation. This flowchart documents the warning signs that preceded Evie's functional seizures and the clinician's interpretation of the warning signs (based on the clinician's knowledge of neurophysiology. © Kasia Kozlowska and Blanche Savage 2022

Once the psychological processes had been identified (see Chapter 8), Evie was able to manage them by using mindfulness-based self-regulation strategies. For example, she now practised noticing and labelling the body sensations, thoughts, and feelings that she was having (in real-time, both in therapy sessions and when warning signs of a functional seizure began to emerge). Next, she practised averting her functional seizure by implementing the neurophysi-ological regulation strategies she had learnt. When she was unable to avert the functional seizure, Evie practised 'surfing the wave' of her body signs, by acknowledging them but also allowing them to rise and fall, knowing that they would pass and that they did not signal something unmanageable or awful.

The therapeutic process of documenting the entire sequence — the somatic warning signs and accompanying self-talk — took several months to develop and address.

For more on 'surfing the wave', see step 4 below and Chapter 10.

```
┌─────────────────────────────────────────────────┐
│      Feeling hot on the outside and cold on the inside     │
└─────────────────────────────────────────────────┘
                          ▼
┌─────────────────────────────────────────────────┐
│  Thinking 'this isn't normal', 'I'm just going to ignore it'  │
└─────────────────────────────────────────────────┘
                          ▼
┌─────────────────────────────────────────────────┐
│  Having tension in the throat (a globus sensation) and an    │
│              unusual taste in her mouth                       │
└─────────────────────────────────────────────────┘
                          ▼
┌─────────────────────────────────────────────────┐
│                  Breathing faster                            │
└─────────────────────────────────────────────────┘
                          ▼
┌─────────────────────────────────────────────────┐
│    Having blurred vision and tingling in the left arm        │
└─────────────────────────────────────────────────┘
                          ▼
┌─────────────────────────────────────────────────┐
│  Thinking 'I am going to push this away', then trying to     │
│         block out any of her bodily sensations               │
└─────────────────────────────────────────────────┘
                          ▼
┌─────────────────────────────────────────────────┐
│              Sharp pain in the chest                         │
└─────────────────────────────────────────────────┘
                          ▼
┌─────────────────────────────────────────────────┐
│  Thinking 'here we go again', 'there's nothing I can do',    │
│  'this is out of my control'; feeling helpless and hopeless  │
└─────────────────────────────────────────────────┘
                          ▼
┌─────────────────────────────────────────────────┐
│           Experiencing a functional seizure                  │
└─────────────────────────────────────────────────┘
```

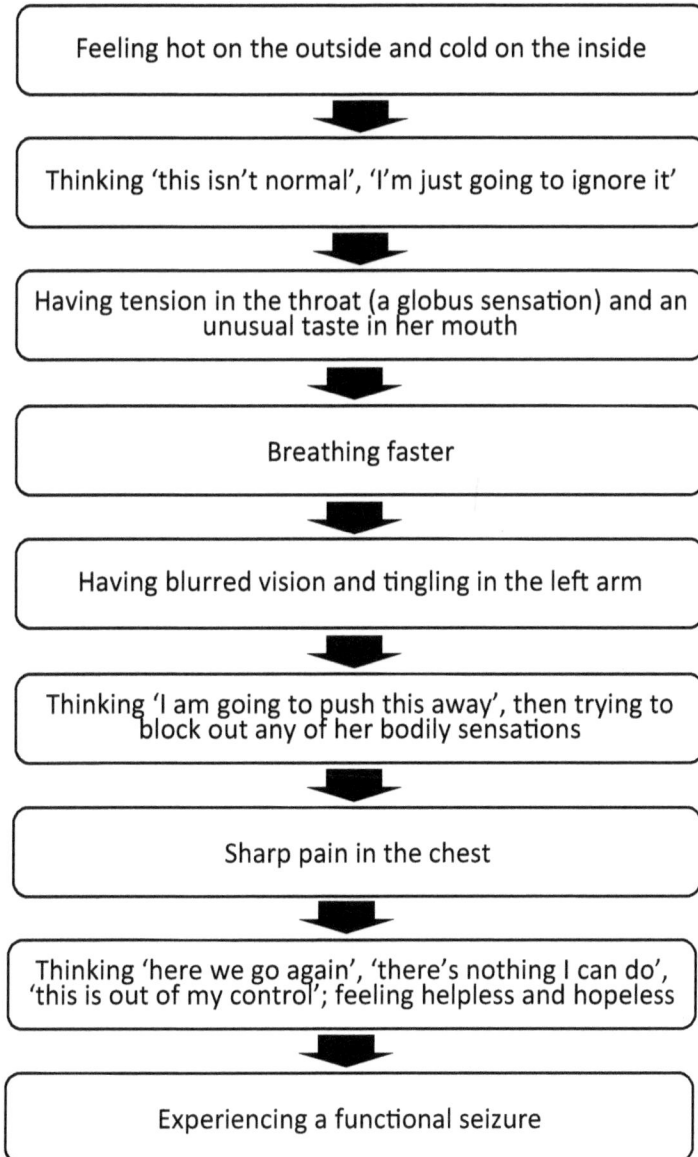

Figure 6.4 Evie's flowchart of warning signs and accompanying thoughts. This flowchart documents the final visual presentation of the sequence of events that preceded Evie's functional seizures: changes in body state (warning signs) and accompanying thoughts and feelings. © Kasia Kozlowska and Blanche Savage 2022

Using Collateral Information

Often parents, caregivers, or schoolteachers will have noticed some of the young person's warning signs (e.g., face going pale, blankly staring, shaking hands, or breathing too quickly). If, as a clinician, you observe the young person having a functional seizure, you may also have observed some warning signs.

For young people who are struggling to recognise their warning signs, access to collateral information may provide you, the clinician, with a starting point for the body map exercise:

> I can see a little shake in your hands. Can you feel that? If you do a quick scan of your body now, is there anything else happening?
>
> or
>
> I can see a little shake in your hands. Can you feel that? I am going to ask you to shift your attention to other parts of the body — just like we practised before — so that we can see what is happening elsewhere in the body. Shall we have a go? Allow your mind to shift your attention to [a body part likely to be involved, such as chest, stomach, muscle region]. Can you tell me what you sense there?

Documenting the Warning Signs of the Five-Step Plan

Once the young person has begun to identify her warning signs, the warning signs should be documented on a visual representation of the Five-Step Plan (see Figure 6.5).[2] Ongoing documentation of the plan — updated as new information comes to be recognised — is important. The plan can be used in hospital settings (e.g., with nursing staff), by the family, and later in the young person's local school.

Because the young person has now begun to identify her warning signs (step 1 of the Five-Step Plan) — or even one or two of her warning signs — you can now begin to work on the next step of the Five-Step Plan (see Figure 6.5).

Step 2 of the Five-Step Plan: Keeping Safe

Because safety is a primary concern for everyone, the second step of any management plan is safety. The young person is asked to sit down or lie down the very moment that she notices any of her warning signs (see Figure 6.5).

The key therapeutic challenge of step 2 is to develop the young person's capacity to shift her focus-of-attention from the felt sense of the body — the

---

2 In ancient Greek mythology, Asclepius was the god of medicine and healing. The rod of Asclepius is a staff with a serpent coiled around it, and it has been used for centuries as a symbol of medicine. The serpent, which sheds its skin regularly, represents rebirth, fertility, and healing. Beginning in the early twentieth century, various medical organisations began using the Caduceus Rod — consisting of two serpents coiled around, usually with wings at the top — as their symbol. We use a stylised version of the Caduceus Rod in Figures 6.5 and 6.6 to provide visual scaffolding for the five steps of the Five-Step Plan. The wavy lines and the steps that they identify represent the progression of the healing process (the process of learning to regulate and gain control over functional seizures), and the wings represent the young person's growing sense of mastery (the capacity to fly).

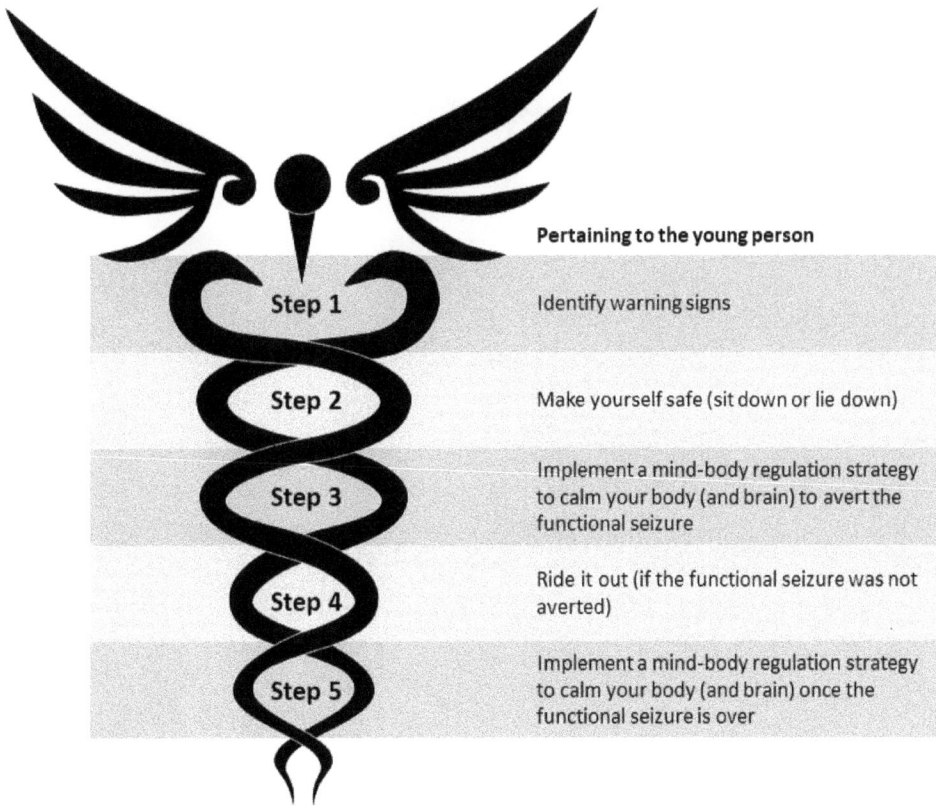

	Pertaining to the young person
Step 1	Identify warning signs
Step 2	Make yourself safe (sit down or lie down)
Step 3	Implement a mind-body regulation strategy to calm your body (and brain) to avert the functional seizure
Step 4	Ride it out (if the functional seizure was not averted)
Step 5	Implement a mind-body regulation strategy to calm your body (and brain) once the functional seizure is over

Figure 6.5 Five-Step Plan for Managing Functional Seizures (pertaining to the young person). © Kasia Kozlowska and Blanche Savage 2022

warning signs of the impending functional seizure — to the behavioural task of getting into a safe position. In so doing, rather than attending to the functional seizure (which she is *not* able to control once it has started), the young person focuses on the task of getting safe (which she *is* able to control). Step 2 not only keeps the young person safe, it shifts the responsibility of staying safe to the young person, and it begins the process of building up her locus of control and mastery — the perception that she has the capacity to control the situation and its outcome.

Step 3 of the Five-Step Plan: Calming the Body (and Brain) Using Mind-Body Regulation Strategies to Avert the Functional Seizure

The clinician and the young person then need to collaboratively decide which mind-body strategies she will use once she is in a safe position (step 3 of the Five-Step Plan; see Figure 6.5). Initially, these may be strategies that distract her attention away from the body, such as listening to music or playing a game on her phone. The expectation is that the young person will develop and add more-targeted strategies to her toolkit over the course of treatment. The clinician should be clear about this expectation with the young person. Step 3 of the Five-Step Plan will be returned to again and again — evolving over the course of treatment as the young person develops new skills.

The overarching goal of step 3 is to avert the functional seizure by interrupting the sequence of activation (see, e.g., the vignette of Evie) — that is, by changing (calming) the body state in the moment. If the young person is successful in using her regulation strategies to avert the functional seizure, she can return to whatever she was doing before she experienced the warning signs.

The key therapeutic ingredient of step 3 is the skill set of mind-body regulation strategies. Bottom-up (body-based) regulation strategies are discussed in Chapter 7, and top-down (cognitive) regulation strategies are discussed in Chapters 9 and 10. Because the brain is part of the body, and because we are using mind-body strategies to calm the brain — as well as the rest of the body — for some young people, it can be helpful to use the term *brain-mind-body strategies*.[3]

Step 4 of the Five-Step Plan: Riding Out the Functional Seizure

If the young person does experience a functional seizure — despite the implementation of her regulation strategies — the plan is to *ride it out* and let the functional seizure take its course (step 4 of the Five-Step Plan; see Figure 6.5).

In our Australian setting, we often use the metaphor of surfing the wave — riding out the functional seizure — because most young people are familiar with the experience of body surfing: catching a wave; losing traction; letting the wave dump you and thrash you around a bit while you hold your breath; swimming back to the surface; beginning all over again (see the surfing-the-wave strategy in Chapter 10). Along the same lines, in Acceptance and Commitment Therapy (ACT), young people are asked to *not fight* unpleasant sensations but to let them come and go (Harris & Hayes, 2007).

Mindfulness skills are the key therapeutic element of step 4. These skills — for any particular patient, at any particular time — may involve forms of bottom-up mindfulness, such as observing and living within the felt sense of the body as the functional seizure comes and passes. Or if that is too difficult, these skills

---

3 We have adopted the term *brain-mind-body strategies* with some of our patients at the suggestion of David Perez and his team at Massachusetts General Hospital in Boston.

may involve forms of top-down mindfulness, such as accepting that functional seizures are not dangerous, that they will come, and that they will pass. Compassion for the self — that is, the recognition that in that particular instance, it was not possible to avert the functional seizure — may also be beneficial. Some young people find it useful to focus on a self-affirming cognition such as 'I can do it' or 'I am safe', which is another top-down (cognitive) regulation strategy or, in the Eastern meditative tradition, a *mantra*.

In practising step 4, the young person needs to accept that she will be successful in averting some functional seizures but not others, regardless of her efforts. The therapist can emphasise that the young person will have many opportunities to practise the task of averting her functional seizures and that eventually she will develop the necessary skills to avert many, and likely even most, of them.

Step 5 of the Five-Step Plan: Calming the Body (and Brain) Using Mind-Body Regulation Strategies After the Functional Seizure

The clinician and young person can also work out what mind-body strategies the young person will implement after the functional seizure to help calm her body (step 5 of the Five-Step Plan; see Figure 6.5). This regulation period should usually be 5–10 minutes of quiet regulating activities. Then the young person should return to whatever she had been doing before the functional seizure.

The overarching goal of step 5 is for the young person to calm her body to a neurophysiological state that optimises her felt sense of wellbeing, her capacity to connect with others (important if the young person is with family or friends), and her capacity to think and learn (important if the young person is at school or at work).

Akin to step 3, mind-body regulation strategies are the key therapeutic element of step 5. Bottom-up (body-based) regulation strategies are discussed in Chapter 7, and top-down (cognitive) regulation strategies are discussed in Chapters 9 and 10.

The Role of the Parent (Supervising Adult) in the Five-Step Plan

Providing parents and other adults with guidelines on how they should respond during a functional seizure should be part of the parent sessions that the clinician runs alongside the young person's sessions (see Figure 6.6 and Chapter 12). Once the parent role is clearly established, it should be included in the management plan. Parents are likely to need coaching to help them respond appropriately to a functional seizure. Key points are the following:

- Functional seizures are not dangerous: they do not cause any injury to the young person's brain.

- It is ultimately going to be the young person's job to monitor and manage her body. As much as parents may want to, they cannot regulate their child's body for her.

- Parents can help their child when she is having a functional seizure by staying calm and in control. If one parent finds it too distressing to be around the young person when she is having a functional seizure, the plan should allow that parent to leave the room while the other parent remains.

- Parents can check that the young person has been able to get herself into a safe position when the functional seizure starts (so that she is unlikely to bang her head or to experience a fall). They can also remind her that she is safe. Once these two things are accomplished, the parents' best approach is to minimise attention to the functional seizure and to monitor the young person from a distance (e.g., in the same room but not right next to the young person). While they are sitting there, the parents can use a regulation strategy (e.g., slow-paced breathing) to calm their own neurophysiological states. If the parents remain calm and show that they are not worried — because their own neurophysiological states are settled — it will help the young person's nervous system calm down faster (also known as *co-regulation*). For additional information about coaching parents, see Chapter 12.

- The young person needs to know that her parents' role is to be quietly present during the functional seizure but not to intervene. Knowing that, the young person will not experience feelings of rejection because the parents have allowed the functional seizure to take its course and have not tried to manage it in an active way.

- The parents should communicate to other adults and children in the young person's life that the Five-Step Plan for the young person *is* the formal management plan for the functional seizures as developed with the young person's treating clinician.

Putting the Five-Step Plan into Picture Form: The Traffic Light Safety Plan for Managing Functional Seizures

The *Traffic Light Safety Plan for Managing Functional Seizures* — for short, Traffic Light Safety Plan — is a visual tool that resonates with younger children and adolescents (see Figure 6.7). The tool translates the information in the Five-

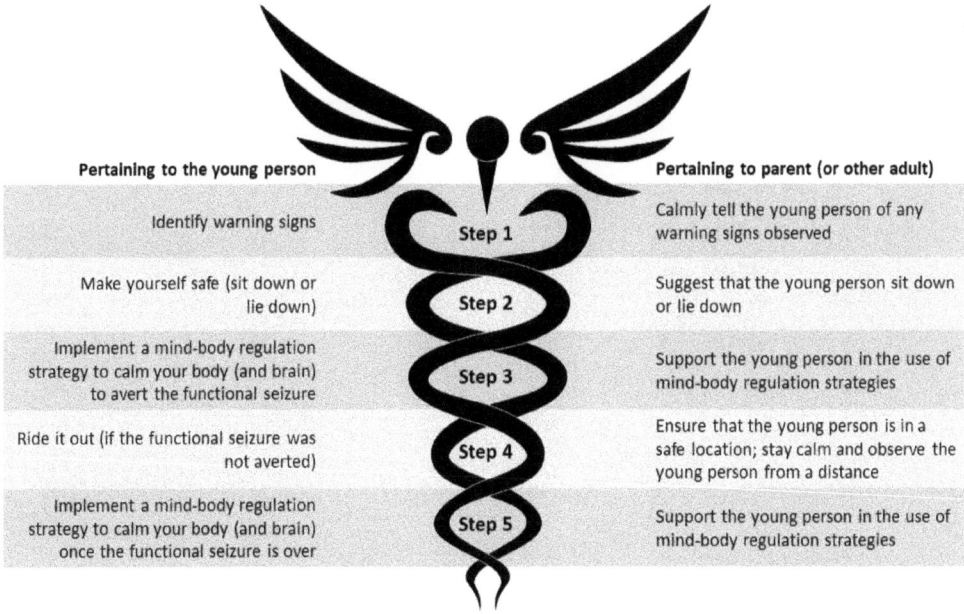

Pertaining to the young person		Pertaining to parent (or other adult)
Identify warning signs	**Step 1**	Calmly tell the young person of any warning signs observed
Make yourself safe (sit down or lie down)	**Step 2**	Suggest that the young person sit down or lie down
Implement a mind-body regulation strategy to calm your body (and brain) to avert the functional seizure	**Step 3**	Support the young person in the use of mind-body regulation strategies
Ride it out (if the functional seizure was not averted)	**Step 4**	Ensure that the young person is in a safe location; stay calm and observe the young person from a distance
Implement a mind-body regulation strategy to calm your body (and brain) once the functional seizure is over	**Step 5**	Support the young person in the use of mind-body regulation strategies

Figure 6.6 Five-Step Plan for Managing Functional Seizures (pertaining to the young person and the parent or supervising adult).
© Kasia Kozlowska and Blanche Savage 2022

Step Plan into a simple picture format, where the five steps are condensed into three colour-coded steps. An added bonus is that parents, grandparents, teachers, and other health clinicians find the Traffic Light Safety Plan easy to understand and use. Blank versions of the Traffic Light Safety Plan — in black and white and in colour, for filling in — are available in Appendix F.

The Traffic Light Safety Plan follows the three colours of traffic lights: green, orange, and red.[4] The green level means that the young person is feeling safe and settled. The orange level is a warning sign that the young person is experiencing the signs of activation and a potential functional seizure. The red level means that the young person is having a functional seizure. For each colour, the young person identifies — with the help of the clinician — all the accompanying bodily sensations, thoughts, feelings, and behaviours. The young person then works out what she should do at that colour level. Some general guidelines for what the young person should do at each step are as follows:

---

4 Some countries (e.g., the United States) may use a green, yellow, and red colour scheme.

Traffic Light Safety Plan for Managing Functional Seizures

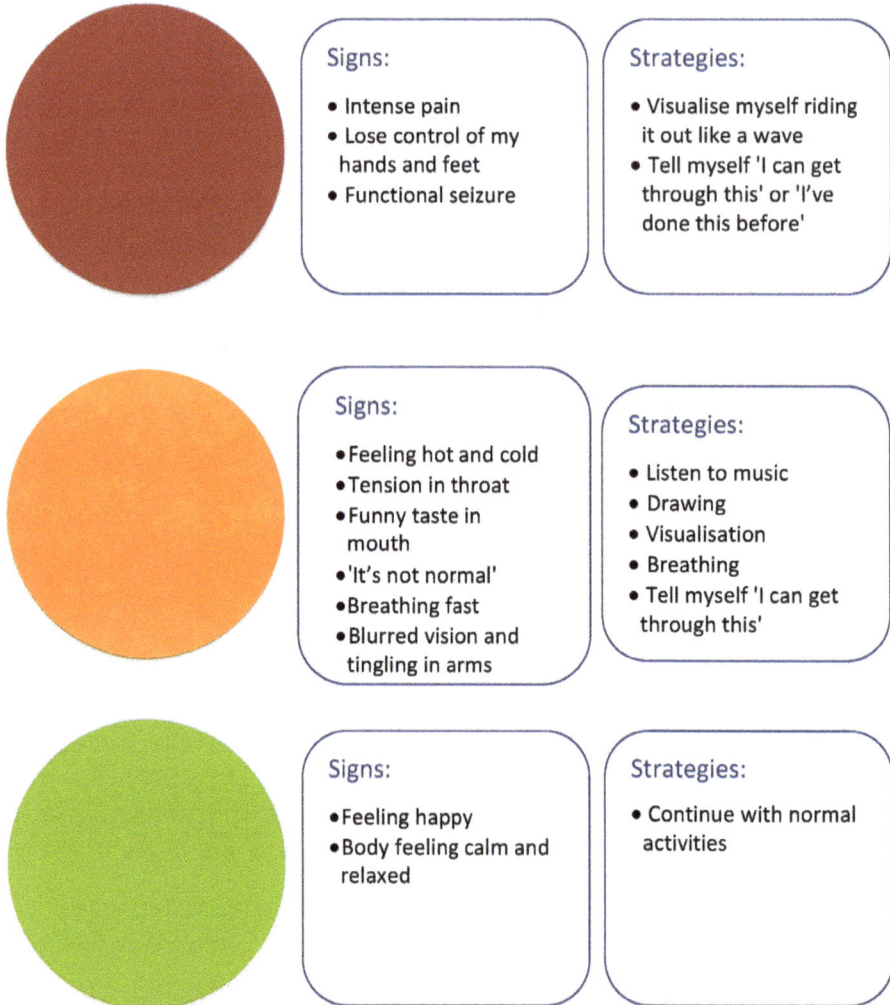

Signs:

- Intense pain
- Lose control of my hands and feet
- Functional seizure

Strategies:

- Visualise myself riding it out like a wave
- Tell myself 'I can get through this' or 'I've done this before'

Signs:

- Feeling hot and cold
- Tension in throat
- Funny taste in mouth
- 'It's not normal'
- Breathing fast
- Blurred vision and tingling in arms

Strategies:

- Listen to music
- Drawing
- Visualisation
- Breathing
- Tell myself 'I can get through this'

Signs:

- Feeling happy
- Body feeling calm and relaxed

Strategies:

- Continue with normal activities

Figure 6.7 Traffic Light Safety Plan for Managing Functional Seizures.
© Danae Laskowski & Kasia Kozlowska 2019

- *Green.* The risk of a functional seizure is low. The young person can continue doing what she is doing.

- *Orange.* The young person is noting the warning signs of a functional seizure and is likely to have a functional seizure (step 1 of the Five-Step Plan). She should sit or lie down on the ground (step 2 of the Five-Step Plan), and she should start using her regulation strategies (step 3 of the Five-Step Plan).

- *Red.* The young person is having a functional seizure, and she needs to 'ride it out' (step 4 of the Five-Step Plan). Any adults present should follow the guidelines outlined in the previous section. When the functional seizure is over, the young person should implement her regulation strategies to calm her body (and brain) (step 5 of the Five-Step Plan).

Troubleshooting

Here we identify some of the common problems that may emerge during the process of developing the Five-Step Plan. We also offer some ideas on how to manage the problems.

- The young person cannot identify any warning signs.

- The young person cannot remember having any functional seizures and therefore cannot remember what the antecedents were for those seizures.

It is often hard for the young person to identify her warning signs. She has, indeed, often spent years dismissing or ignoring what her body is signalling. The task of 'reading her body' is therefore a new skill for her to learn. If the young person cannot identify her warning signs, talk to her about this being a new skill that she is learning. Make a positive prediction that she will, with practice, learn and even master this skill. If the young person remains sceptical or resistant, do not focus on her inability to identify warning signs or push her further to identify them. Instead, leave spaces in subsequent therapy sessions for the young person to add warning signs to her Five-Step Plan if she begins to identify them. For example, check in regularly to ask the young person whether she has noticed any more warning signs; or if the young person starts to talk about a recent functional seizure, ask whether she noticed any warning signs beforehand; and so on.

If you and the young person are really stuck, you may need to engage in elemental work about listening to the body — that is, in noticing and tracking the felt sense of the body. For example, you and the young person can practise the body scan exercise (see Chapter 7) to help her build skills in reading her body. One possibility is to practise the exercise as part of progressive muscle relaxation, encouraging the young person to tell the differences in muscle tension before, during, and after tensing. You can also activate the body via movement or laughter and support the young person in attending to how her body feels before, during, and after any of these activities.

If you and the young person continue to be stuck, it can be helpful to normalise her difficulties in reading the body — for example, 'It is very tricky to read the body. A lot of young people with functional seizures find reading the body difficult.' — and to engage in some additional simple psychoeducation. As one possibility, the metaphor of the autonomic nervous system (see Figure 4.3) can be used to discuss the body in a calm state (the blue on the picture) and an activated state (the red on the picture). The clinician can say, 'When the red system switches on, the heart can start to pound, our breathing can become faster, and our muscles can become tense. Have you noticed any of these things happening in your body?'

Further complications:

- The young person cannot use any strategies even if she identifies her warning signs.
- The young person says that none of the strategies are helpful.
- The strategies do not work straight away.
- The young person refuses to try any strategies.

Remind the young person that if she wants to reduce or avoid her functional seizures, she will need to use and practise her regulation strategies. Remind parents, caregivers, and other professionals involved in the case (e.g., teachers) that nobody can make a young person learn to regulate her body. The role of adults is to encourage and support this skill-based learning process. If the young person makes the choice not to learn, practise, or use any strategies, acknowledge that this means that she will continue to have functional seizures. But also make a positive prediction that she will still be able to learn the strategies in the future — when she is ready. For now, you should focus on ways to help her *ride out* the functional seizures (step 4 of the Five-Step Plan), and you should make suggestions as to what she can do after a functional seizure occurs to help her body return to a better-regulated state (step 5 of the Five-Step Plan).

Chapter 7

Working with the Body: Neurophysiological (Bottom-Up) Regulation Approaches

Functional seizures present in and through the body, and for that reason, our mind-body team has found that interventions that target the body have an inherent acceptability for young people and their families. In the current literature this group of interventions is known by a variety of names, including *bottom-up regulation approaches, neurophysiological regulation, body-oriented psychotherapy, sensorimotor psychotherapy, somatic experiencing, therapeutic touch, body mindfulness, bottom-up mindfulness,* and *biofeedback interventions* (Bloch-Atefi & Smith, 2015; Cristea et al., 2021; Kain & Terrell, 2018; Ogden & Fisher, 2015; Payne et al., 2015). In the clinical setting, therapists who use neurophysiological (bottom-up) regulation often use 'shorthand' to refer to these interventions. For example, they may refer to 'settling' or 'calming' the young person's 'nervous system' or simply to 'calming the body down'.

The Aim of Neurophysiological (Bottom-Up) Regulation Approaches

The aim of neurophysiological regulation is to help the young person regulate her body state[1] — including the brain — to promote synchrony, harmony, and balance within and between body systems, as well as 'the efficient flow and utilisation of energy' (McCraty & Childre, 2010, p. 18). Figure 7.1 depicts two body maps drawn by an adolescent girl — one depicting her body state before a session on neurophysiological regulation and one depicting her body state after the session.

---

1 As noted in earlier chapters, because functional somatic symptoms occur more frequently in girls than in boys, we generally use the pronouns she and her to reflect this clinical reality.

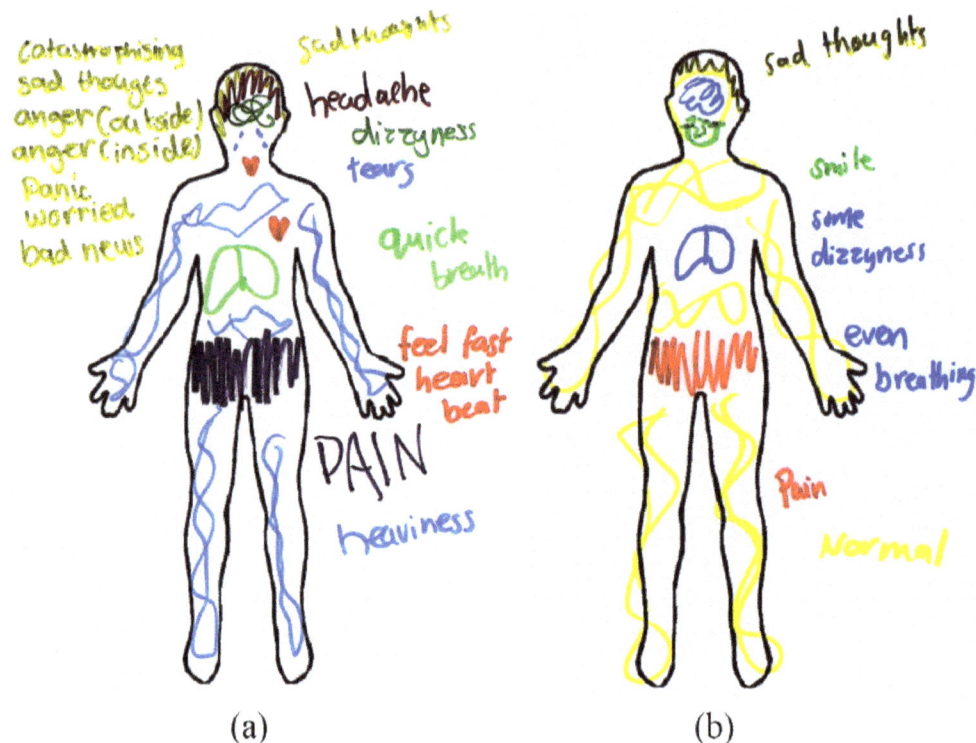

Figure 7.1 Body maps before and after a therapy session. These body maps are the work of an adolescent girl. (a) The first body map depicts the girl's body state at the beginning of a therapy session, when she is in a highly aroused state. (b) The second map depicts the shift in the girl's body state at the end of a therapy session in which the girl completed a training session in neurophysiological regulation — using a slow-breathing intervention with biofeedback — followed by a relaxation exercise with soothing imagery. © Kasia Kozlowska 2018

To regulate body state is to achieve a balance within a set of overlapping and interrelated hormonal, neural (autonomic nervous system), immune-inflammatory, and brain systems that make up the body's stress system (see Figure 1.3). The stress system mediates the brain-body stress response, including the body's ability to regulate itself and its use of energy in response to the challenges of daily life.

As we saw in Chapters 4 and 6, young people with functional seizures typically experience a state of stress-related high arousal — involving the activation of body systems — prior to their functional seizures. And as described in detail in Chapter 1, this activation, of necessity, requires a high use of energy, whereas states of active engagement (with lower levels of stress) involve a middle range of energy use, neither too high nor too low.[2] Daniel Siegel uses the term window of tolerance to refer to neurophysiological states in which arousal is neither too high nor too low (Siegel, 1999). These matters are crucial for understanding functional seizures. Current research suggests that young people with functional seizures may activate neural (brain) networks to such an extent that these networks become unstable when faced with perturbations in energy flow, as in the case of additional demands for energy associated with stress, new threats, or perceived threats or stress (Radmanesh et al., 2020). That is, when the energy demands reach biological limits, neural networks may dysregulate, resulting in a functional seizure.

Neurophysiological (Bottom-Up) Regulation Calms the Body in the Moment

Neurophysiological regulation strategies change body state and, in particular, calm the body even as they are being implemented. They can be used by the young person to calm her body in the moment — that is, as soon as she perceives her body state to be activating or perceives the warning signs of a functional seizure. Given that functional seizures reflect a state of temporary activation and dysregulation within neural networks, they are incompatible with a state of neurophysiological regulation — that is, with body states that sit within the window of tolerance. Functional seizures are much less likely to occur if the young person (over time and through repeated practice) is able to achieve and maintain herself in a state of relative calm.

In addition, once the young person has achieved some degree of neurophysiological regulation using bottom-up strategies, she will be in a better position to try using top-down cognitive strategies (see Chapters 9 and 10). These top-down strategies engage the prefrontal cortex and are difficult to implement whenever prefrontal cortex function is disrupted by stress-related changes associated with a state of neurophysiological activation and dysregulation (Arnsten, 2015).

Consequently, when treating functional seizures, our mind-body team generally starts with bottom-up (body) regulation strategies before moving to top-down (mind or cognitive) strategies. Cognitive strategies work better when the body (including brain) is relatively settled.

---

2 For more detail about energy regulation, including the role of the hypothalamic-pituitary-adrenal (HPA) axis and the autonomic nervous system, see Chapters 6 and 8 in Kozlowska, Scher, and Helgeland (2020) and articles by Kleckner and colleagues (2017) and Jungilligens and colleagues (2022).

Setting Up Expectations About the Process of Neurophysiological (Bottom-Up) Regulation

How the clinician sets up expectations in relation to this component of treatment is very important. Our team tries to set the following expectation for the young person:

> We are going to explore a whole range of different strategies to
> help your body calm down. Most young people don't like
> everything we try, but everyone finds a few strategies that help
> them. It will be interesting to see which strategies you like to
> work with.

Our aim as clinicians is to trial different neurophysiological regulation strategies in therapy sessions and for the young person to practise the ones she regularly likes throughout the week. We encourage practising regulation strategies four times a day for five minutes and also every time the young person notices the warning signs of a functional seizure (her body becoming activated). We emphasise that it is important to practise these strategies when feeling calm and settled so that the young person can use them effectively when she is feeling aroused/activated. The practice of regulation strategies should be added to the young person's daily timetable that the clinician has begun to develop collaboratively with the young person and the family (see Chapter 5). The regulation strategies should also be added to the young person's Five-Step Plan (see Figure 7.2 for an updated timetable and also Chapter 6). As noted earlier, visual representations of the Five-Step Plan are available in Appendix C (for the young person) and Appendix D (for the young person and parent [or other adult]). Both are suitable for printing, and translations of Appendixes C and D into some other languages are available online from the publisher.

Neurophysiological (Bottom-Up) Regulation Strategies and Functional Seizures

The Body Map: Listening to the Body and Reading the Warning Signs of an Impending Functional Seizure

Listening to the body's somatic narrative — and being able to read the state of the body — is the first step in implementing neurophysiological regulation approaches. In the scientific literature, the somatic narrative — 'the sense of the physiological condition of the body' (Craig, 2003a, p. 500) — is referred to as *interoception, homeostatic feelings, homeostatic emotions, neuroception,* and *bottom-up mindfulness* (Craig, 2003b; Guendelman et al., 2017; Kabat-Zinn, 2003; Kozlowska, 2013; Pace-Schott et al., 2019; Porges, 2009).

7.00 am to 7.30 am	Wake up Practise slow breathing in bed before getting up
7.30 am to 8.00 am	Breakfast, get dressed, get ready for the day
8.00 am to 9.00 am	Leave for school Listen to playlist of 'happy music' in car on the way to school
9.00 am to 3.00 pm	School (Eat morning tea and lunch) Take stress ball & fidget toys into school to use in class
3.00 pm to 4.00 pm	Practise grounding strategies in car on the way home from school
4.00 pm to 4.30 pm	Afternoon tea Practise slow breathing
4.30 pm to 5.00 pm	Half an hour of exercise with mum (for example, walk the dog, jump on trampoline, or go for a swim)
5.00 pm to 6.00 pm	Homework (Monday, Tuesday, Wednesday) Gymnastics (Thursday) Youth group (Friday)
6.00 pm to 7.30 pm	Free time
7.30 pm to 8.00 pm	Dinner
8.00 pm to 8.30 pm	Free time
8.30 pm to 9.30 pm	Start bedtime routine: Move phone out of room and log off any devices Have a cup of herbal tea Have a warm shower Practise slow breathing Read in bed
9:30 pm	Lights out and sleep

Figure 7.2 Updated timetable that supports daily rhythms and that includes body regulation strategies.

When the body activates — increases its level of arousal — there are multiple changes throughout the body (see Figure 7.3).

Visual representation	Clinical sign or symptom (felt sense of the body)	Biological process
	Increased heart rate	Withdrawal of parasympathetic activity ± increased sympathetic activation
	Breathing faster	Respiration becomes more rapid due to activation of the motor-respiratory system
	Feeling sweaty	Sweat gland secretion increases due to activation of the sympathetic system
	Dry mouth	Saliva production decreases because sympathetic activation causes vasoconstriction of blood vessels that supply the salivary glands
	Dilated pupils or widening of the eyes	Sympathetic activation of the pupil
	Tense or high-pitched voice	Tone in the proximal laryngeal (striatal) muscles increases
	Knotted stomach	Tone in smooth muscles (e.g., the stomach) increases
	Tension in the body	Tone in all other striated muscles and the fascial tissue that supports them — and especially those involved in posture — increases

Figure 7.3 Common signs and symptoms associated with increased arousal.
© Kasia Kozlowska 2019

If the young person has developed the skill of listening to the body, many of these neurophysiological changes can be experienced subjectively. Young people commonly report a range of somatic markers, including the following: thumping heart; rapid breathing; sweatiness or a sudden change in temperature; dry mouth; tightness in the throat or chest; tightness or butterflies in the gut; and tension — or even pain — in the head, neck, back, or muscles of the legs.

In our work with young people, we ask them to draw their body state on a body map (see Chapter 6 and Figure 6.1). This visual depiction makes the somatic narrative more concrete and easier for the young person and clinician to keep in mind. With time and practice, young people become more skilled at listening to their bodies and reading their warning signs of a functional seizure. They will also learn to implement regulation strategies as soon as they detect the body's signals that an increase in arousal/activation — the warning signs of a functional seizure — is taking place.

Breathing Strategies (Slow-Paced Breathing)

The neural networks regulating breathing and the neural networks regulating the autonomic nervous system (arousal) are *coupled systems*. They are located close to each other in the brain stem, and they work together in a synchronised way (Benarroch, 2007; Lamotte et al., 2021). What we see in clinical practice — and especially with young people with functional seizures — is that increases in arousal are often accompanied by increases in breathing rate. When the breathing rate is greater than metabolic demand — the body's energy needs —

it is called *hyperventilation*. This coupling is important from a therapeutic perspective: the young person can utilise slow-paced breathing to down-regulate (calm down) the autonomic nervous system (Gerritsen & Band, 2018).

Hyperventilation activates neural networks; that is, it increases neural network activity and brain arousal.[3] Young people with functional seizures frequently hyperventilate, and for some individuals, hyperventilation can trigger a functional seizure (Kozlowska, Rampersad, et al., 2017). This is because young people with functional seizures activate the neural networks with hyperventilation but are then unable to down-regulate them back to normal (Braun et al., 2021). Put simply, the brain stays in an activated state for a prolonged period of time. Text Box 7.1 shows common signs or symptoms (felt sense of the body) that are caused by hyperventilation. Because many children trigger their functional seizures by hyperventilation, many of the warning signs of increased

---

Text Box 7.1
Common Signs and Symptoms (Felt Sense of the Body) Caused by Hyperventilation

Caused by neurophysiological changes in the brain

- Blurring of vision, an experience of colours, or blackout
- Buzzing in the head
- Dizziness, light-headedness, giddiness or faintness, sensations of unreality or floating, loss of consciousness, or fainting (all reflecting varying degrees of reduction in the level of consciousness)
- Increased anxiety, panic, weeping, and various emotional reactions reflecting a loss of top-down inhibition

Caused by neurophysiological changes in the peripheral nervous system

- Numbness and tingling of the hands, feet, and face
- Tension of stiffness of the muscles (e.g., tense band across the head)
- Severe cramping in the hands and feet (called *tetany* in medical circles)

Caused by imbalance of blood gasses

- Feeling of breathlessness, smothering, not getting enough air (air hunger)
- Chest pain (caused by narrowing of arteries to the heart due to hypocapnia)
- Excessive sighing or yawning

Caused by high use of energy and concomitant increase in sympathetic arousal

- Fatigue
- Dry mouth (increase in sympathetic arousal)

---

3 For the neurophysiology of hyperventilation, see Online Supplement 7.1 of Kozlowska, Scher, and Helgeland (2020).

activation — and an impending functional seizure — are the body's response to hyperventilation.[4]

It can be helpful to measure the young person's breathing rate at rest (i.e., how many breaths she takes in a minute). A relaxed child in the resting state should breathe 7–21 times per minute, and a relaxed adolescent in the resting state should breathe 7–18 times per minute. Anything over this reflects a high respiratory rate (>75th percentile) and is a sign that the stress system is switched on and that the young person's body is in a state of overactivation. Clinically, it can be difficult to notice hyperventilation unless you count the breathing rate.

Begin by introducing slow, diaphragmatic breathing (belly breathing). This is the first step because individuals who hyperventilate often breathe by using the intercostal muscles (between the ribs) more than the diaphragm. Ask the young person to lie down and place something on her stomach (a cup or a toy). The goal is for the young person to make the item rise and fall with her breathing. Ask her to breathe into the bottom of her lungs first. This step can take some practice before the young person is able to breathe primarily using her diaphragm. Once the young person has mastered this, coach her to slow down her breathing. Initially, aim for 5–10 breaths slower than her resting breathing rate (e.g., if the young person's resting breathing rate is 30 breaths per minute, coach her to breathe at 20 breaths per minute). The young person should practise this 3–4 times a day. After this target breathing rate has been achieved, see if the young person can further slow her breathing rate. The ideal breathing rate for calming the body (increasing restorative parasympathetic function) is 6–8 breaths per minute. However, many young people with functional seizures need extensive practice to achieve that level.

For some young people, changing their breathing rates can feel uncomfortable, and a small number complain of dizziness. We explain to young people that these symptoms are a sign of the body recalibrating to breathing at a slower rate and that the symptoms will settle over time and practice. For this reason, it is better for young people to gradually reduce their relaxed breathing rates over a number of weeks. This is also the reason we encourage young people to initially practise slow breathing while lying down.

A handful of young people are unable to utilise slow-breathing interventions because focusing attention on breathing — and any attempt to control breathing — will trigger a panic attack and an increase in breathing rate. In that

---

4 For more detail see Engel and colleagues (1947) (a landmark study of hyperventilation), Online Supplement 7.1 of Kozlowska, Scher, and Helgeland (2020), and Sawchuk and colleagues (2020).

scenario, alternative strategies that do not focus on the breath — but that slow down the young person's breathing rate indirectly (such as hypnosis or guided imagery) — need to be pursued (see Chapters 9 and 10).

Many online resources are available to help individuals — including younger children — practise slow-paced breathing (e.g., variations of breathing exercises [Shakeshaft, 2012] or Youtube videos on five-finger meditation for children). Some resources provide information on the use of props (e.g., bubbles or feathers) to help children to learn to regulate breathing. Other options include the use of humming, bee breathing, box breathing, or the *voo* sound (Brown & Gerbarg, 2005; Cleveland Clinic, 2021; Levine, 2010).

Biofeedback

Heart rate variability (HRV) is the variation in time between heartbeats. HRV can be used as a proxy measure of the body's stress system and specifically the autonomic nervous system. When you are relaxed — activating the calming (parasympathetic) component of the autonomic nervous system — your HRV is relatively high. When you are stressed — you have switched off the calming component of the autonomic nervous system and may be switching on its activating (sympathetic) component — your HRV is reduced. A number of biofeedback programs have been developed to help people improve their HRV by regulating their breathing. These programs measure a person's HRV and coach the person on breathing exercises to decrease the respiratory rate and calm the body, resulting in a measurable increase in HRV. Some of these apps can be used on smartphones or other devices.

In this rapidly changing field of biofeedback, technology is evolving quickly. In the past, our team has used apps such as HeartMath, Heart Rate + Coherence Pro, and IOM2, each of which has advantages and disadvantages. We would suggest that you, the clinician, look at what is available at the time you are using this manual, with these three apps being a potential starting point. Importantly, not all biofeedback devices used in clinical practice are of adequate quality for research (Rajabalee et al., 2022).

Grounding Strategies

By connecting the young person physically to the present moment, grounding strategies can help her feel contained when she is feeling overwhelmed by states of high arousal or strong emotions. Grounding strategies are implemented by asking the young person to use each of her senses to focus on the present moment. For example, you can ask the young person to feel and describe the feeling of her feet on the floor, the chair pressing into her back, the colours of objects in the room, or the sounds that she hears. Likewise, the *five senses grounding strategy* is a helpful way to support the young person in connecting to her body — and sense of embodied self — using all the sensory modalities (sight, touch, hearing, smell, and taste). This strategy involves asking the young person to identify five things she sees, four things she feels, three things she hears, two things she smells, and one thing she tastes (Lozier, 2018). Grounding strategies can be helpful during times of high arousal/distress as a way of supporting the young person to shift her focus-of-attention away from sensations from within the body (and associated with activation/arousal) to sensations from outside the body (and associated with calm and safety). Mental health clinicians trained in Dialectical Behaviour Therapy (DBT) will have been taught some commonly used grounding strategies to help highly aroused young people avoid becoming overwhelmed — strategies often referred to as TIPP skills (Temperature [e.g., use of ice], Intense exercise, Paced breathing, and Paired muscle relaxation) (Rathus & Miller, 2002).

Therapeutic Touch

Some young people are able to use therapeutic touch to help themselves settle. For example, a hand on each shoulder — in a self-hug — can be calming. A hand on the chest, accompanied by humming or the humming of a tune can be calming. Another strategy that some young people find regulating is to have a hand on the heart and a hand on the back of the neck and to rock gently backward and forward. The clinician and young person will have to experiment with different strategies in session to find the one that the young person finds calming. Therapeutic touch is a core element of somatic experiencing and sensorimotor psychotherapy (see below for references for further reading).

Therapeutic touch can also be helpful when a young person's breathing pattern is dysregulated — for example, if she is holding her breath, breathing irregularly, or breathing in a jerky fashion. In such cases, it may be calming for the parent or clinician to put a hand on the young person's shoulder and remind her out loud, 'You are safe. Let your breath go all the way down to your tummy.'

Body Scan

The body scan — from the Eastern tradition of mindfulness meditation (Kabat-Zinn, 1982) — is particularly useful for young people who disconnect from their body sensations or their emotions as a coping strategy. The body scan exercise is used to support the young person's connection and awareness of her body state by focusing attention on different body parts. It can also help support a young person learning to shift her attention from body sensations of activation/arousal to a part of the body that feels calmer. Initially, the body scan is done as a therapist-guided activity, where the therapist leads the young person to focus on sensations through different body parts (often starting from the head and working down to the feet). The body scan can be done at different paces, depending on the aim — for example, doing the body scan slowly to induce a state of calmness and bottom-up mindfulness, or at a more rapid pace to support the young person in connecting with her physical and emotional state. Various apps are available.

As with the slow-breathing strategies outlined above, a small number of young people find that in paying attention to body state, they become fixated on sensations of neurophysiological activation and cannot shift their attention away, leading to an escalation of neurophysiological activation that may culminate in a panic attack or a functional seizure. This experience can be a useful demonstration of how unhelpful it is to focus and attend to body symptoms; for these young people, alternative regulation strategies may need to be trialled. With time, after they have learnt the skill of shifting attention, these young persons may be more successful at utilising the body scan.

Progressive Muscle Relaxation

Progressive muscle relaxation is a helpful intervention for young people who are holding a lot of tension in their bodies without being aware that they are doing so. It can both help to increase young persons' awareness of their body states and also help them to activate states of calm. Progressive muscle relaxation, which can be considered an extension of the body scan, requires the young person to focus on different body parts and then to relax them. The exercise can be done by tensing different muscle groups and letting the tension go, or by just noticing muscle tension and letting it go. For young people with chronic pain, tensing of the muscles may not be appropriate; only the latter (i.e., noticing muscle tension and letting go) should be used. Various apps are available.

Sensory Tools

Some young people, especially when other strategies seem ineffective, may respond well to the sensory input provided by sensory tools. If your service has access to occupational therapists, they can be particularly helpful at helping young people find sensory tools that work for them. Otherwise, the clinician and family can trial different strategies to find what works best for the young person.

Sensory tools that help some young people calm their bodies include the following:

- Weighted blanket or weighted toys
- Body sock or compression clothing
- Fidget toys
- Slime/putty
- Stress balls

- Stroking or spending time with a pet
- Sucking on sour lollies
- Holding ice
- Chewing gum
- Smelling calming scents (e.g., a scented candle or essential oils)
- Listening to music
- Looking at photos of nature
- Making and using a mindfulness glitter calm down jar. The young person shakes the jar and watches its contents slowly settle (Kumarah Yoga, 2022).

For younger children, these strategies can be put together into a sensory box. Ideally, the sensory box should incorporate something for all five senses (sight, touch, hearing, smell, taste) and be something that the young person can access easily.

Movement Interventions

Movement interventions — including physical exercise — have a wide-ranging, modulating impact on neuroendocrine and other physiological systems, and can be used as bottom-up regulation strategies in their own right (Kim et al., 2021; Rosenwinkel et al., 2001; Shafir, 2016). Movement interventions have an important role in addressing autonomic dysregulation, increasing resilience and stress resistance, and activating a complex set of mechanisms that promote neuroprotection (Kim et al., 2021). Repetitive movements are particularly important in helping to regulate emotions and the stress system (Shafir, 2016).

Examples of movement interventions include the following:

- Sitting and bouncing on a gym ball
- Lying on your tummy on a gym ball and rocking backward and forward
- Rolling a gym ball backward and forward with another person (either sitting or standing)
- Swinging on a swing
- Rocking in a rocking chair
- Rocking, swaying, or gently bouncing
- Jumping on a trampoline

- Drumming
- Ping-pong, shooting hoops, bouncing balls, handball, and so on
- Swimming
- Cycling
- Using a rowing machine
- Rhythmically tensing and releasing your thigh muscles
- Stamping your feet rhythmically, or tapping on your legs in a regular pattern or to music

Music as a Regulation Intervention

Both listening to and producing music can be calming activities for young people; these activities engage sensorimotor, cognitive, and emotional processes (Vuilleumier & Trost, 2015). Music (potentially under the guidance of a music therapist) can be used as a regulation strategy in a number of ways:

- The young person can choose musical tracks that activate positive feeling states that are incompatible with states of distress and high arousal. She can divert attention to the music when she notices her warning signs of brain-body activation.

- Alternatively, the young person can create a playlist of music — ideally, music that has 60 beats a minute — or access an available list that research has found to be helpful for neurophysiological regulation (Saarman, 2006; University of Nevada Reno Counseling Services, n.d.). See also Safe and Sound Protocol in the next section.

- A parent can — with previous negotiation — play chosen music tracks during or following a functional seizure to help the young person in her task of regulating body state.

- Music can be combined with movement (e.g., dance or drumming), and the two together can be integrated into the young person's day as a regulation strategy.

- Singing or humming has potential value as a regulation strategy. For some young people, singing along loudly to a favourite song helps to distract them from paying attention to their body symptoms. For other young people, singing or humming helps them regulate their breathing and down-regulate their bodies.

- Some young people choose to write music or play an instrument as a way of processing and conveying emotional states that they may not be able to communicate effectively through talking alone.

Other Neurophysiological (Bottom-Up) Regulation Interventions That Can Be Delivered by a Trained Practitioner

- *Safe and Sound Protocol.* This music-based neuromodulation intervention was developed by Stephen Porges (Porges, 2018; Rajabalee et al., 2022). It is a passive, bottom-up regulation intervention that involves listening to five hours of music that is designed to help regulate the autonomic nervous system. The Safe and Sound Protocol can be used as an adjunct to other therapeutic interventions. Research studies looking at its efficacy are pending.

- *Somatic experiencing and sensorimotor psychotherapy.* Practitioners trained in somatic experiencing and sensorimotor psychotherapy use a broad range of bottom-up interventions. They work with the felt sense of the body, careful directing of attention (bottom-up mindfulness), breath work, therapeutic touch, movement (e.g., Smovey rings), and so on. See, for example, the work of Peter Levine, Kathy Kain, Patricia Ogden, and Abi Blakeslee (Blakeslee, 2021; Kain & Terrell, 2018; Levine, 2010; Ogden & Fisher, 2015).

- *Massage.* See, for example, slow-stroke massage (Arnold et al., 2020; Baumgart et al., 2020).

Integrating Bottom-Up Regulation Strategies into the Timetable

Once young persons have some regulation strategies that they can use, they need to practise them regularly throughout the day — and as noted above, with practice times integrated into the daily schedule (see Figure 7.2).

Chapter 8

Working with the Mind I: Identifying Illness-Promoting Psychological Processes

This chapter — the first of three chapters about *working with the mind* — is largely theoretical. We use the chapter to introduce you, the clinician, to the illness-promoting psychological processes that our mind-body team commonly sees in young people with functional seizures. Because our work with young people with functional seizures has evolved in the context of neuroscience research, we use Antonio Damasio's neuroscience framework regarding emotions, feelings, and thoughts (Damasio & Carvalho, 2013; Damasio, 1994). In this framework, the term *emotion* is used to describe a body state (e.g., the body state of being hurt or being afraid) and the word *feeling* is used to describe the subjective experience of that body state (e.g., feeling pain or feeling afraid). In Damasio's framework, feelings sit alongside thoughts to make up a young person's mental life. Thoughts include word images, picture images, sound images, olfactory images, tactile images, and images pertaining to body state (Damasio, 2018). Feelings and thoughts evolved because they help keep us alive: they 'constitute a crucial component of the mechanisms of life regulation, from simple to complex' (Damasio & Carvalho, 2013, p. 143). We find this framework especially useful because it highlights the importance of both bottom-up and top-down processes — and the interaction between them — in our subjective experience of emotions (our feelings). It also sees human consciousness as grounded in biological processes (Damasio, 1994; Pace-Schott et al., 2019; Jungilligens et al., 2022), which we think is important for understanding the interconnection between mind and body.

Here we note — for the benefit of clinicians who are trained in traditional cognitive-behavioural therapy (CBT) — that Damasio's framework is very different from the CBT framework of behaviour, thoughts (including physical sensations that are elicited by certain thoughts), and feelings. Damasio's framework emphasises bottom-up processing. Changes in body state occur in the body itself; this information about body state is provided to the brain on a second-by-second basis; and some of these body states become available to subjective experience in the form of feelings (e.g., feeling pain [a homeostatic feeling] or feeling afraid). The CBT framework emphasises top-down processing (i.e., the mental generation of thoughts and feelings) and the physical sensations that might accompany particular thoughts and feelings (i.e., the body's response to the thoughts or feelings). See Chapter 10 and Text Box 10.1 — the Three Waves of Cognitive-Behavioural Therapy — for a discussion of how CBT has evolved over the last century (Brown et al., 2011; Hayes, 2004; Hayes & Hofmann, 2018).

In contrast to this chapter, which is theory laden, the two chapters that follow are clinically oriented. Chapter 9 discusses focus-of-attention and the important role of expectations pertaining to the therapy. Chapter 9 also addresses the manner in which the skill of shifting focus-of-attention is integrated into the Five-Step Plan (see Chapter 6). Chapter 10 discusses therapeutic options that can be used to manage illness-promoting psychological processes — focusing on cognitive (top-down) regulation strategies — and the manner in which cognitive strategies can be integrated into the Five-Step Plan (see Chapter 6).

As noted earlier, visual representations of the Five-Step Plan are available in Appendix C (for the young person) and Appendix D (for the young person and parent [or other adult]). Both are suitable for printing, and translations of Appendixes C and D into some other languages are available online from the publisher.

The Role of the Human Mind in Activating and Calming the Stress System

The human mind is a powerful tool, and the young person can use it to activate or calm the stress system. The young person's mental life, like that of adults, includes a vast array of mental processes, including all her feelings and thoughts[1] — whether thinking in words or concepts, or about events (real or imagined, internal or external, or past, present, or future), or through feelings representing the state of the body (e.g., feeling fatigued, feeling hungry, feeling breathless [air hunger]).[2] Whatever the source, all these psychological processes

---

1 As noted in earlier chapters, because functional somatic symptoms occur more frequently in girls than in boys, we generally use the pronouns she and her to reflect this clinical reality.

2 The feeling of breathlessness — of not getting enough air (air hunger) — is a common symptom of hyperventilation (see Text Box 7.1).

and the associated images emerge from within, as part of the young person's inner mental life, and the brain interprets and appraises them in the same way that it appraises images generated by external stimuli (Damasio, 1994; Gianaros & Wager, 2015; Jungilligens et al., 2022). If the feelings or thoughts are interpreted and appraised as threatening, brain-body pathways linking psychological stress and the neurophysiological state of the body are activated, switching on the stress system via top-down mechanisms (Gianaros & Wager, 2015) (see Figure 8.1). For example, the event of witnessing a car crash and the subsequent mental event of remembering the car crash will both activate the stress system. In this way, the feelings and thoughts generated by the human mind can, in and of themselves, function as cognitive stressors.

Put simply, thoughts and feelings pertaining to danger, fear, anger, rejection, and disconnection up-regulate (activate) the stress system, whereas thoughts and feelings pertaining to safety, joy, goodwill, connection, acceptance, and so on down-regulate (calm) the stress system. So, if the young person with functional seizures trains her mind to recognise and acknowledge difficult, dangerous, and unpleasant thoughts but then moves on to focus on those that are calming, her cognitions will contribute to the healing process and the maintenance of ongoing health and wellbeing. If, by contrast, she dwells on the

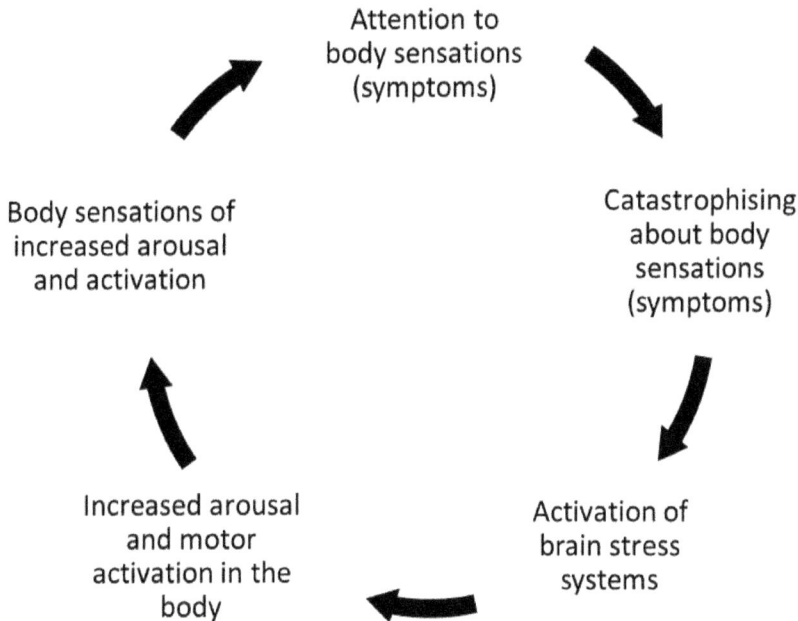

Figure 8.1 Vicious cycle metaphor. The figure depicts an example of a vicious cycle — one that includes illness-promoting thoughts — that can be part of the clinical presentation. © Kasia Kozlowska and Blanche Savage 2022

thoughts pertaining to danger, fear, and so on, her cognitions will contribute to stress-system activation and the processes that drive her functional seizures (and any comorbid functional neurological symptoms). Illness-promoting psychological processes are also common with anxiety and depression (Beck, 1976; Hummel et al., 2021).

An important point in this context is that in some cases, the thoughts and feelings pertaining to danger, fear, rejection, and so on are the product of the young person's lived experience in the here and now: the danger, fear, or rejection is real. If so, the situation needs to be recognised and addressed in order to protect the young person.

Why Is Identification of Psychological Processes So Important?

It is our observation that illness-promoting psychological processes are often under-recognised by health professionals. Identification of such psychological processes is not part of the *neurology* assessment for functional seizures. And within the *mental health setting*, efforts to identify illness-promoting psychological processes are typically embedded within the assessment of anxiety, depression, or other mental health disorders. If the young person does not meet diagnostic criteria — or does not present with symptoms of anxiety, depression, or other formal mental health disorder — further efforts to explore illness-promoting psychological processes may not be undertaken. The upshot is that illness-promoting psychological processes will often remain unrecognised and unaddressed, and continue to contribute to symptom generation and perpetuation. See Text Box 8.1.

In the three vignettes below, we see the powerful role that cognitive processes can have in triggering or maintaining functional seizures and why the content of this theory-laden chapter is so important in learning to work with young people with functional seizures.

Text Box 8.1
A Key Learning Point About Identifying and Addressing Psychological Processes

Being able to identify and address psychological processes is an important element of working with the young person with functional seizures — of working with the mind. Illness-promoting psychological processes can block the young person's recovery if not addressed. Such processes contribute to both the vulnerability to functional seizures (and other somatic symptoms) and the persistence of symptoms, and can block constructive treatment processes.

A 13-year-old adolescent girl wanted to become a doctor. Her expectations pertaining to her grades at school were exceedingly high. She had decided that any test score less than 90% was unacceptable. When she failed to perform to the expected level, she experienced negative cognitions — for example, intrusive thoughts of 'This is because I didn't try hard enough,' 'I've really let my parents and my teachers down,' and 'I'm a fraud and not really as smart as people think.' These thoughts were followed by obsessive rumination about all the things that she could have done differently in order to have received a higher score — 'if only I hadn't seen my friends yesterday' and 'if only I'd stayed up later to study longer' — and they were coupled with intense feelings of distress. On many occasions these thoughts and feelings generated states of overwhelming arousal, culminating in functional seizures in the school classroom.

Another adolescent stated, 'I got a 94% on a science test,' and his automatic thought was, 'What happened to the other 6%? What did I get wrong?'

BJ, a 16-year-old boy, experienced vivid intrusive flashbacks of physical and emotional abuse from his father.[3] Daytime flashbacks triggered functional seizures that presented in one of three ways: faint-like episodes, faint-like episodes followed by violent jerking of limbs, or faint-like episodes followed by a long period of unresponsiveness.

Centrally Important Psychological Processes: Focus-of-Attention and Expectations of the Treatment Process

Two psychological processes — attention to symptoms and the formation of expectations about the therapeutic process — have a role in shaping the treatment course and outcome of all young people presenting with functional seizures. These processes must be taken into account and addressed across all system levels (the family, all components of the medical system, and the school) and in all five steps of the Five-Step Plan (see Chapter 6).

Attention to Symptoms

Attention 'is the taking possession by the mind, in clear and vivid form, of one out of what seem several simultaneously possible objects or trains of thought' (James, 1890, pp. 403–404).

---

3 BJ's case history has been reported in detail in Ratnamohan and colleagues (2018).

Attention to functional somatic symptoms amplifies the symptoms, and attention away from the symptoms diminishes them (see Text Box 8.2). For this reason, managing focus-of-attention is a key element of the therapeutic process. The manner in which you, the clinician, manage focus-of-attention across treatment interventions and across system levels will play a central role in achieving and maintaining progress. Likewise, the manner in which the young person and the family learn to respond to the young person's symptoms — how she directs her focus-of-attention — will help determine the symptoms' ongoing significance in the young person's life. And, of course, because it is your job to help the young person and family accomplish this therapeutic task, you need to have a good understanding of focus-of-attention and how to manage it. In Chapter 9 we examine focus-of-attention in greater detail.

Expectations

Expectations — the young person's thoughts and beliefs about what will happen in the future — are also very powerful. Expectations shape — at least in part — the manner in which the brain processes a broad range of sensory, motor, interoceptive, and emotion-related information (Edwards et al., 2012; Kleckner et al., 2017). Expectations about the therapeutic process channel the young person's footsteps onto a path of health and wellbeing or, alternatively, onto a path of ill health and disability (see Text Box 8.3).

For example, a young person who expects an intervention (including medication) to have therapeutic effect is more likely to experience some of those effects. This is called the *placebo effect*; it activates health-related and

---

Text Box 8.2
A Key Learning Point About Attention

Attention to symptoms — by the young person, the parents, or health care clinicians — worsens functional neurological symptoms (including functional seizures) and amplifies subjective pain.

Text Box 8.3
A Key Learning Point About the Power of Positive Expectations

Positive expectations harness the healing elements of treatment interventions: they diminish activation of the brain stress systems and the severity of functional somatic symptoms (including comorbid pain).

---

healing neural pathways. By contrast, when a young person expects an intervention to be unhelpful or likely to cause side effects, she is likely to experience minimal therapeutic effects and more adverse effects. This is called the *nocebo effect*; it activates illness-related neural pathways. The shaping of the young person's (and family's) expectations is consequently an important component across therapeutic interventions (Benedetti, 2013; Wager & Atlas, 2015). For this very reason, throughout this manual we regularly remind you, the clinician, of the importance of setting up positive expectations that will help steer the therapeutic process toward a good outcome.

Negative expectations (nocebo effect) can be established and maintained in a number of ways. They can emerge as part of the young person's 'catastrophic symptom expectations' (Fobian et al., 2020) or her thoughts and feelings associated with a low sense of control over her symptoms (see sections below). They can also be influenced by the beliefs and behaviours of parents, clinicians, and school staff.

Negative expectations, particularly around illness beliefs and the potential for recovery (or lack thereof), can undermine the efficacy of strategies that the young person needs to learn to manage the symptoms. Common examples of this process include the following:

'I've tried breathing before. It didn't help.'

'Nothing is going to work.'

'This is not real treatment.'

'If relaxation strategies helped, that would just prove it was all in my head.'

An adolescent girl believed that the Mind-Body Program was a form of 'torture'. She declined to come into the program — preferring, in effect, the path of chronic illness, with the consequence that she remained wheelchair-bound.

An adolescent girl believed that medications were bad for the body. When medication for depression was trialled, she experienced myriad side effects.

A school-age boy experienced side effects as soon as he took his prescribed medication (from the time that the medication was in his mouth or just swallowed [i.e., not yet digested]).

A mother was certain that her 12-year-old son would not be able to bear being apart from her in hospital. She said repeatedly (in front of her son) that he would be too anxious and too sad. When she tried to leave the bedside, the son had repeated panic attacks and functional seizures.

In this context it is the clinician's task to set up positive expectations in an ongoing way (see Chapter 9).

Illness-Promoting Cognitive Processes Pertaining to the Functional Symptoms Themselves

Because you, the clinician, have already spent time working and talking with the young person, you are probably already beginning to identify some of the psychological processes — specific to that young person — that may be relevant contributing factors. Our aim in this section of the chapter is to discuss a broad range of psychological processes so that you, the clinician, can recognise them as they arise. In some young people, one or more of these psychological processes can be so powerful that they can function as *roadblocks* to clinical progress and lead to symptom perpetuation. Hence the therapeutic goal of identifying these processes (this chapter) and addressing them (Chapters 9 and 10) is very important. Here we begin by discussing illness-promoting cognitive processes that pertain to the functional symptoms themselves.

Catastrophic Symptom Expectations

To *catastrophise* means thinking about the worst possible outcome of an action or an event. Catastrophic symptom expectations are thoughts that the symptoms will eventually lead to catastrophic outcomes. Examples of this process include the following:

> An adolescent girl presented with functional seizures and motor symptoms. It was a challenge to manage her catastrophic symptom expectations. In response to a new pattern of pain, the girl's thoughts ran as follows: 'What is wrong now? How bad is it going to get?' These thoughts were coupled with a mental image of her body shaking and going into a functional seizure.

> An 11-year-old adolescent girl with functional seizures, loss of motor function, and allodynia in the right leg held a belief that the water in the hydrotherapy pool would press against her leg and cause her excruciating pain. She believed that the pain would be worse at the deep end of the pool because it was filled with more water. It took months before she would allow her foot to be submersed at the shallow end of the pool. And it was months more before she felt comfortable at the deep end. In the interim, she experienced pain during all her hydrotherapy sessions and communicated this by high-

pitched screams. Frequently, the pool session would be ended by a prolonged functional seizure.

An adolescent girl presented with functional seizures, leg weakness, and pain that kept her legs in a bent position all the time. She reported minimal pain when in the hydrotherapy pool — where her legs straightened without any conscious effort. When encouraged to straighten her legs in her bed, she often refused, foreseeing that the pain would be excruciating (catastrophic symptom expectation). At the mere suggestion of straightening her legs, the girl would become tense and grimace.

Misinterpreting the Body and Its Signals

Some young people with functional seizures lose track of what body signals are normal and which are not.

During the morning ward round, an adolescent girl told her treating team that something was wrong with her bladder because she was not going to the bathroom to urinate hourly — as she usually did. Her team replied that this was wonderful news. Her body was finally learning to regulate itself; most girls her age went to the bathroom to urinate 2–3 times in a morning. Her irritable bladder was finally settling down, as were her functional seizures. The girl's functional seizures began to settle as soon as she had acquired the skills needed to manage her focus-of-attention (see focus-of-attention in the Five-Step Plan [Chapters 6 and 9]).

Low Sense of Control over Symptoms

The lack of control over symptoms — the difficulty of predicting how and when the functional seizures will emerge, especially prior to treatment — can leave a young person feeling helpless, activate the stress system, and undercut efforts to move forward in treatment.

'My symptoms happen out of the blue.'

'This [sudden sharp pain in chest] sucks. I am better off dead.'

'I don't get any warning signs. The next thing I know I am lying on the ground.'

Illness-Promoting Cognitive Processes Pertaining to Life Challenges in General

We continue the chapter by discussing cognitive processes that are not directly related to the functional somatic symptoms but that function to promote the illness process various ways, including as cognitive stressors that switch on the stress system via top-down mechanisms (Gianaros & Wager, 2015) and as beliefs and expectations that block some element of the therapeutic process, thereby contributing to symptom generation and maintenance.

Catastrophic Thinking Pertaining to the Self and to the Non-Self

Catastrophic thinking can also pertain to the self or to a broad range of situations, including, for example, the environmental challenges confronting the earth itself. This thinking is typically coupled with feeling overwhelmed, which in turn can exacerbate symptoms.

> 'If I don't get everything correct [on the upcoming test], I'll never be able to become a surgeon.'

> 'When the glacier melts, we won't have any water, and we'll all die.'

Low Sense of Control Regarding Events or Expectations in the Home or School Setting

The young person may have recurrent thoughts that reinforce a perceived lack of control regarding events or expectations in the home or school setting. Such thoughts are usually coupled with feelings of helplessness.

> 'It's too hard. I can't do it. I hate school.'

> 'They all think I am stupid.'

Perfectionistic Thinking

Perfectionistic thinking raises expectations in relation to commonplace life responsibilities, and it demands that the young person maintain such high levels of performance that the expectations become a source of stress in and of themselves.

> 'I did not reply to my brother's text because I could not get my text right.'

> 'I only got 98% in the math exam' [associated with a feeling of disappointment and sadness]. In one adolescent girl, this thought alone — coupled with her continuous state of high arousal — was enough to trigger a functional seizure.

Self-Critical Rumination

Rumination involves obsessive negative or distressing thoughts about an idea, situation, or choice. Self-critical rumination refers to the process of berating oneself regarding what one could or should have done. When talking with young people, we sometimes refer to self-critical rumination as beat-yourself-up thoughts.

> 'I didn't try hard enough [to get well]. It is my fault I am back in hospital. I should have tried harder and done better.'

> 'The money my parents are spending on my treatment means my family is missing out.'

> 'Only weak people have anxiety. The [treatment] team must think I'm really weak to suggest I have anxiety.'

Obsessive Thinking

Obsessive thinking refers to the inability to switch thought processes away from a certain idea or worry. In addition to being an independent source of stress, obsessive thoughts take up a lot of energy and mental space, preventing the young person from focusing on tasks that have therapeutic value.

> An adolescent girl, hospitalised for treatment of functional seizures, was obsessed with the accuracy of her diagnosis. Each morning at ward rounds she grilled her team about her diagnosis, including the pros and cons of formally including other diagnoses on her chart in addition to functional neurological disorder (FND): fibromyalgia, postural orthostatic tachycardia syndrome, complex/chronic pain, irritable bowel syndrome, and so on.

Mental Rigidity (Black-and-White Thinking)

Black-and-white thinking refers to thinking in absolutes.

> A teenage girl could not let go of the idea that the actions of her mother, who had recently been somewhat critical of her school grades, were the sole cause of her functional seizures. The intervention included psychoeducation about the many different factors that contributed to functional seizures, along with mediation sessions between the girl and her mother — leading the mother to apologise and, as reported by the rest of the family, to work hard to change her parenting style. Nevertheless, the teenager could not move on from the idea that her functional seizures were all her mother's fault. She returned to this idea again and again (obsessive thinking, see above).

> An adolescent boy hospitalised for functional seizures believed he could only return to school once his functional seizures had fully resolved. He stated, in a very emphatic way, 'You go to school when you are well and stay home when you are unwell.' To assist the adolescent, the clinician spent time discussing the importance of *working toward wellness* when treating functional disorders. The clinician explained that with many other medical diagnoses, the normal course of action was get well *before* returning to school. But with functional disorders, going to school and engaging in normal activities — while still unwell — were part of the treatment. To assist the adolescent with this challenge, a graded return-to-school plan was developed collaboratively (see Chapter 13).

Negative Focus Regarding the Future, Coupled with the Inability to Be in the Present

An exclusively negative focus regarding the future, coupled with the inability to be in the present and to celebrate progress in the here and now, is sometimes seen.

> An adolescent girl who had presented with leg paralysis, cognitive impairment, and functional seizures complained that everything was getting worse and that her occasional drop attacks made life impossible. She forgot to mention — or celebrate — that she was now dancing around the house and that her cognitive capacities had returned.

Feeling-Related Processes

Feeling Overly Responsible

Some young people have caregiving roles in their family or in the school setting. In the context of this role, they feel overly responsible for the welfare of others. They often feel compelled to act as confidants and mediators in relationships. In such circumstances the weight of the responsibility is more than the young person can manage, contributing to stress-system activation and to the presentation of functional seizures.

> An adolescent girl was very attuned to the distress of others within her friendship group at school and felt it was her responsibility to settle distress felt by others or to sort out disputes between friends.

> An adolescent boy, the second eldest in the family, felt it was his responsibility to keep younger siblings safe while an older sibling with autism was out of control or while his parents were fighting.

Lingering Negative Feelings: Worry, Sadness, Anger, Guilt, Helplessness, Hopelessness

Pervasive negative feelings that come up in the young person's mind time and time again are common but might not meet the diagnostic criteria for anxiety or depression. They can include any of the following:

> Chronic worries about schoolwork, friendships, or parental wellbeing
>
> Experiencing sadness or a low mood but not being able to admit and share these feelings with attachment figures
>
> Experiencing anger but not being able to admit or share these feelings
>
> Feeling guilt about asking for help, about feeling sad or worried, or for taking up a hospital bed
>
> Feelings of hopelessness that are associated with cognitions such as 'Nothing will work ... There's no point trying.'

Pushing Difficult Thoughts Out of Mind (Cognitive Avoidance)

Attempting to manage worries and difficult thoughts — and the associated emotions — by pushing them out of mind is a common coping strategy. Though this strategy is sometimes helpful in the short term, when it persists, it prevents the young person from grappling with issues that need to be addressed.

> An adolescent girl did not tick the questionnaire item pertaining to family conflict. When asked why, she explained that her father — with whom she was in sharp conflict — was no longer part of her family.

Pushing Difficult Feelings Out of Mind (Feeling Avoidance)

Some young people manage uncomfortable or unpleasant feelings (e.g., grief, worry, sadness, or anger) by blocking them out of their minds — that is, by pushing them away and trying not to feel them. In a parallel process they also disconnect from unpleasant body states associated with strong emotions (feelings being the subjective experience of those emotions). In young people with functional seizures (and other FND symptoms), the most common scenario is to have feelings of anger that are pushed out of mind. Research data from assessments of attachment suggest that in this group of young people and their families, the overt expression of anger is seen as an unacceptable emotion within the family system (Kozlowska et al., 2011).

> When a clinician asked an adolescent boy with functional motor weakness and functional seizures about the potential impact of his parent's separation, the boy replied, 'Nah, it's fine.'

Fear and Avoidance of Activities

Fear and avoidance of activities — including school — are commonly seen in young people with functional seizures. This unfortunately places the young person in a typical anxiety feedback loop, whereby avoiding the activity makes it harder to return to the activity and succeed at it, and consequently increases the anxiety/arousal (and likelihood of having a functional seizure).

> An adolescent boy had come to fear and avoid exercise because it exacerbated his pain and triggered autonomic system activation that resulted in panic attacks or functional seizures.

> An adolescent boy was unable to cope with the high academic expectations in his school setting. During the time that he attended the hospital school, he was able to engage in schoolwork that had been sent by his local school. When he returned to the local school — following his discharge — he was unable to manage the same work. He became overwhelmed and told the teacher that the work was too hard.

Disconnecting from the Felt Sense of the Body (Subjective Awareness of Body States)

In Chapter 7 we discussed the idea of the felt sense of the body — that is, the subjective awareness of body state. The felt sense of the body includes homeostatic feelings (e.g., thirst, itch, pain, and fatigue) and also higher-order feelings associated with the basic emotions (e.g., happiness, sadness, fear, anger, surprise, and disgust). Young people with functional seizures not uncommonly disconnect from body states: changes in body state are difficult for them to notice and track, and the task of learning to read the felt sense of the body is a serious challenge. This disconnection has implications with regard to the young person recognising warning symptoms, in the form of body sensations, of an impending functional seizure.

> An adolescent girl with functional seizures had no subjective awareness that she was breathing at 45 breaths per minute. She had also ignored the frequent butterflies in the stomach, the changes in tension in the

muscles of her neck and back, and the band of pain across her forehead — which signalled activation of her body stress systems.

An adolescent with leg weakness, panic attacks, and functional seizures regularly insisted that she loved school and that she did not find school to be stressful. Notwithstanding, she experienced a relapse of symptoms every time reintegration to school was attempted despite being symptom-free in hospital.

An adolescent girl pushed herself relentlessly in her effort to achieve at school and to fulfil her role as peacemaker within her friendship group. She overrode all warning signs — disrupted sleep, headaches, dysregulated gut, extreme fatigue, and intrusive thoughts of self-harm — that she was pushing her body too much. Eventually, her punishing schedule was forcibly disrupted when she developed functional seizures (and a myriad of other functional neurological symptoms). Throughout the treatment process, the task of finding the healthy middle way — expectations of herself that were not too much and not too little, based on what her body could manage — was an ongoing challenge.

An adolescent girl was so disconnected from her body states that she was unable to tell when she was hungry. Her food intake was based on time of day and never on any cues of hunger.

Attachment-Related Processes

Inability to Seek Comfort and Protection from Attachment Figures

The core element of balanced (secure) attachment is the capacity to seek comfort and protection from the attachment figure when experiencing stress, illness, or threat to one's safety or psychological integrity. Examples of at-risk (non-secure) patterns of attachment include the following: being unable to tell parents that not all is well; not telling parents about what is happening so that the young person protects (does not burden) her parents; and not being able to ask parents for help. Research studies have found that it is common for both children and adults with FND to show at-risk (non-secure) patterns of attachment (Asadi-Pooya et al., 2021; Kozlowska et al., 2011).

A school-age girl was not able to tell her parents about her feelings of sadness or anger, or about the experience of being worried and overwhelmed. When she was with them, she laughed and smiled and worked hard to maintain an external facade of being okay.

A school-age boy did not tell his parents about bullying and, instead, tried — unsuccessfully — to manage it all by himself in an effort to protect his parents from becoming too stressed.

An adolescent girl began to struggle with the academic demands — particularly with mathematics — on transition to high school. She did not signal her difficulties to her parents, and she was unable to ask her teacher for help, thereby perpetuating problems at school and the subjective stress that she experienced.

Amplifying Signals of Distress to Activate Caregiving Behaviour from Parents and Others

An alternate strategy seen in at-risk (non-secure) patterns of attachment is an amplification of signals of distress to activate caregiving behaviour from parents, teachers, health staff, and so on. In some families, although it is not acceptable to signal *emotional distress*, communication of unpleasant homeostatic, physically oriented feelings (e.g., pain or fatigue) may be permitted.

A boy with an abnormal gait coupled with back pain signalled his pain via loud, lingering wails as he laboriously made his way to the hospital's schoolroom.

Evie, an adolescent girl experienced prolonged functional seizures at school preceded by sharp pains in the chest; when she experienced this sequence of events, she would scream out that she was dying and ask why no one was helping her.

Loss, Trauma, and Other Adverse Experiences

Within an attachment framework, lack of resolution of loss, trauma, and other adverse experiences refers to a maladaptive psychological response to a dangerous or threatening event that continues to adversely affect the young person's functioning in the here and now (Crittenden & Landini, 2011; Farnfield et al., 2010).

In this scenario the young person may be preoccupied with the traumatic, unresolved event, which may be a frequent element of her mental life: her thoughts, memories, and feelings. Alternatively, the young person may block the event out of mind. In this scenario memories and feelings are omitted from mind and from the young person's narrative. Intermittently, however, they may come into the young person's mind unbidden (intrusively).

When unresolved experiences are identified as a key element of the presentation for functional seizures, trauma-focused work — radical exposure tapping (MacKinnon, 2014), eye movement desensitisation and reprocessing (Pagani et al., 2015), trauma-focused CBT (Cohen et al., 2012), and so on — may need to be started. Trauma work typically also requires work with the family. It is common for trauma to remain unresolved because the family has not provided the young person with the opportunity to talk about or process the event and to form an integrated understanding of the trauma (which would include experiencing a body state that is settled when the trauma comes to mind).

> An adolescent girl presented with multiple FND episodes. Each was triggered around the anniversary of her father's past hospitalisation — when her father had almost died.
>
> Another adolescent girl, Xenia — now living with her grandparents — had been exposed to significant family stress from three years of age (Xenia's co-constructed formulation was discussed in Chapter 3). At certain points in her developmental history, she and her siblings had suffered from neglect, including insufficient food coupled with the lack of appropriate adult presence and supervision. At other times she had witnessed significant domestic violence and had been concerned about the safety of her mother, her siblings, and her own self. After moving to live with her grandparents, the girl had been able to push these memories out of mind. A photo of one of the perpetrators in the newspaper had triggered trauma-related memories. The memories emerged — night after night — in the form of nightmares. Three weeks later, a netball injury triggered a cascade of functional symptoms: leg weakness, nausea, dizziness, and functional seizures presenting as blackouts.

Checklist of Illness-Promoting Psychological Processes

We end this chapter by providing you, the clinician, with a checklist of psychological processes. The checklist (Figure 8.2) is a handy tool that can remind us of the broad range of illness-promoting psychological processes that may need to be addressed (see Chapter 9).

Psychological process	Process present
Centrally important psychological processes	
Attention to symptoms	
Negative (vs. positive) expectations pertaining to treatment interventions	
Illness-promoting cognitive processes pertaining to the functional symptoms themselves	
Catastrophic symptom expectations	
Misinterpreting the body and its signals	
Low sense of control over symptoms	
Illness-promoting cognitive processes pertaining to life challenges in general	
Catastrophic thinking pertaining to the self and non-self	
Low sense of control regarding events or expectations in the home or school setting	
Perfectionistic thinking	
Self-critical rumination (beat-yourself-up thoughts)	
Obsessive thinking	
Mental rigidity (black-and-white thinking)	
Negative focus regarding the future (± inability to be in the present)	
Feeling-related processes	
Feeling overly responsible	
Lingering negative feelings: worry, sadness, anger, guilt, helplessness, hopelessness	
Pushing difficult thoughts out of mind (cognitive avoidance)	
Pushing difficult feelings out of mind (feeling avoidance)	
Fear and avoidance of activities (activity avoidance)	
Disconnecting from the felt sense of the body (subjective awareness of body states)	
Processes related to attachment, family, and relationships	
Inability to seek comfort and protection from attachment figures	
Amplifying signals of distress to activate caregiving behaviour from others	
Unresolved loss, trauma, and other adverse experiences	

Figure 8.2 Psychological process checklist.
© Kasia Kozlowska and Blanche Savage 2021

Working with the Mind II: Focus-of-Attention and Expectations of the Illness Process

In Chapter 8 we noted that some psychological processes — attention to symptoms and expectations about the therapeutic process — are so common that working with them is always part of the therapeutic intervention. In this chapter we discuss these two issues in more detail. From your perspective as the clinician, your skill set in managing focus-of-attention and supporting positive expectations across treatment interventions and across system levels will play a central role in achieving and maintaining progress. From the perspective of the young person, her skill[1] in shifting focus-of-attention and her capacity to maintain positive expectations become core elements of the Five-Step Plan (see Chapter 6). In order for the young person and the family to engage successfully in the therapeutic process involving focus-of-attention, they need, more broadly, both to understand and be confident in the treatment plan.

As noted earlier, visual representations of the Five-Step Plan are available in Appendix C (for the young person) and Appendix D (for the young person and parent [or other adult]). Both are suitable for printing, and translations of Appendixes C and D into some other languages are available online from the publisher.

Managing Attention Across the Therapy Process: A Key Challenge for the Clinician

As a starting point, it is helpful to understand the changing manner in which focus-of-attention needs to be managed at different time points in the

---

1 As noted in earlier chapters, because functional somatic symptoms occur more frequently in girls than in boys, we generally use the pronouns she and her to reflect this clinical reality.

Text Box 9.1
Working with Focus-of-Attention

Attention to symptoms — by the young person, the parents, health care clinicians, or school staff — worsens functional neurological symptoms (including functional seizures) and amplifies subjective pain. In this context, focus-of-attention needs to be carefully managed in health care settings, at school, and at home.

---

therapeutic process. Because this process is complicated, and because you, the clinician, need to take charge of the process, it is helpful to consider focus-of-attention across the three key phases of the therapy.

Phase 1: Focus-of-attention during the assessment process

The assessment process is the only phase of treatment where focus-of-attention is on the symptoms themselves. During the assessment, you, the clinician, will (inescapably) be paying attention to symptoms as you put together a comprehensive story exploring how they arose and as you acknowledge and validate them as real, distressing, and disabling. At this point in the therapeutic process — the process of engagement — it is very important that you validate and acknowledge the young person's experience because many young people report that their symptoms and experience of the symptoms have been dismissed by other clinicians.[2]

Phase 2: Focus-of-attention during the formulation process and during psychoeducation

At the end of the assessment process — at which point you will co-construct the formulation that has emerged from the family's story (see Chapter 3) — and again during psychoeducation (see Chapter 4), you will highlight that attention amplifies symptoms, and you will be putting the family on notice that learning to manage attention away from symptoms will be a core element of all treatment components. In doing so, you are already shifting focus-of-attention away from the symptoms themselves to the treatment interventions that the young person and family will learn in order to manage them.

---

2 For a detailed account of patient stories of unhelpful interactions within the medical system, see Kozlowska and colleagues (2021).

Phase 3: Focus-of-attention during the treatment intervention(s)

Once the treatment process has begun, you (the clinician) and all the members of the multidisciplinary team will support the young person (and family) — over and over again, in each component of the treatment intervention — in practising the task of shifting attention away from the symptoms. The challenge is to maintain a balance between acknowledging the young person's experience (to avoid re-enacting previous interactions where the young person has been dismissed or ignored) and shifting attention away from the symptoms. The clearer that one is in phases 1 and 2 about the importance of shifting focus-of-attention, the easier this challenge becomes during the treatment itself (phase 3).

To illustrate this point, here we briefly describe how the multidisciplinary team in our Mind-Body Program manages focus-of-attention in every component of the treatment intervention. On morning rounds — the first scheduled event of the day — our focus-of-attention is on the day's timetable and on the young person's efforts to practise her regulation strategies the previous day, evening, and night (not on the symptoms themselves). Therapy sessions focus on attaining skills to manage the symptoms (not on the symptoms themselves). In the hospital school, focus-of-attention is on engaging in school activities and on learning (not on the symptoms). In physiotherapy, managing focus-of-attention away from symptoms is a core element of the Wellness Approach to physiotherapy for young people with functional neurological disorder (FND), including functional seizures (Gray et al., 2020; Kim et al., 2021). And we remind you, the clinician, that regular pleasurable exercise is part of the daily timetable for every young person with FND (including functional seizures) (see Chapter 5).

As Part of the Five-Step Plan: A Key Challenge for the Young Person

Most young people require significant coaching and support to become adept at implementing the focus-of-attention element of the intervention. Our mind-body team has found that some young people find it helpful when we discuss focus-of-attention explicitly across the five steps of the Five-Step Plan.

Focus-of-attention during each step of the Five-Step Plan is as follows:

Step 1: Focus-of-attention on the warning signs of a functional seizure

The young person needs to direct her attention to the felt sense of the body (emerging symptom pattern) — what we call the *warning signs* — that inform her that her body is activating (see Chapters 6 and 7).

Step 2: Focus-of-attention on the task of assuming a safe position

The young person needs to shift her attention away from the felt sense of the body (emerging symptom pattern) to the behavioural process of getting herself into a safe position on the ground (so that she does not fall and cannot injure herself).

Step 3: Focus-of-attention on the regulation strategy

Once safe on the ground, the young person needs to shift focus-of-attention to the process of implementing a regulation strategy to calm her body and to derail the emerging symptom pattern (to avert the functional seizure).

Step 4: Focus-of-attention on riding it out

If the young person has not been able to avert the functional seizure, the young person needs to acknowledge this fact, and she needs to shift focus-of-attention to the task of riding it out — that is, letting the body do its thing (activate and then settle down). During this process many young people find it helpful to shift focus-of-attention via a preprepared script (e.g., 'It is OK. I can do it.') or, alternatively, to shift focus-of-attention onto a guided visualisation exercise (in recorded form) or music track, which their parent may facilitate via the use of earphones.

Step 5: Focus-of-attention on the regulation strategy

As soon as the functional seizure is over, the young person needs to shift focus-of-attention to the process of implementing a regulation strategy to calm her brain and body to a state that is not compatible with experiencing another functional seizure, and that will allow her to get on with her daily activities.

In Relation to Pain and Other Functional Symptoms:
A Key Challenge for Everyone

Many young people with functional seizures also suffer from comorbid pain and other functional somatic symptoms (including nausea, fatigue, dizziness, and motor and sensory symptoms) (see Figure 1.1). In treatment, these young people learn to manage focus-of-attention in relation to all of these symptoms; that is, they practise the skill of drawing focus-of attention away from all functional symptoms and onto the tasks of the day. For an in-depth description of how this is achieved during physiotherapy sessions, see Gray and colleagues (2020) and Kim and colleagues (2021).

A Key Challenge for the Family

Managing focus-of-attention when working with the family — the family system level — is likewise a core element of the treatment process. Attention to symptoms often occurs — via verbal, visual, or motor-sensory cues — in the context of day-to-day interactions between the young person and the family. Many of these processes are quite subtle and are not always easy to identify.

> The young person's mother focused her gaze on her son every time he got up to move around the room.

> The child's mother soothed the child's brow — stroking it over and over again — following each functional seizure.

> The child's father checked in about how the child was feeling — including the level of pain and nausea — many times a day.

> The mother of Nina, an adolescent girl, checked in daily, first thing in the morning, to see whether Nina was well enough to go to school. Nina consequently started attending to her body and searching for any potential symptoms from the time she woke up. And by searching for such symptoms, she increased the likelihood of finding some. When speaking with Nina's parents, the clinician acknowledged that they were caring and attentive. The clinician highlighted that this was usually a very good thing but that in this particular situation, it was too much of a good thing. It drew Nina's attention to her symptoms and amplified them. Nina's mother became distressed and asked why no one had given her this information before.

Once some of the attention-related interactions have been identified, the clinician will need to support the family in practising how to redirect focus-of-attention on health-promoting behaviours and interactions. Importantly, if this family component is not addressed — for whatever reason — the probability of future relapse is increased. In our own hospital-based setting, we highlight this point to families by emphasising that during the admission, they — the families — are building up a skill base that will enable them to take the Mind-Body Program home. The skill of managing focus-of-attention in a way that does not perpetuate functional seizures — and other functional somatic symptoms — is part of this skill base. Chapters 9 and 10 discuss this work with the family in more detail.

In Other Settings

The clinician may also need to address focus-of-attention in other medical and social settings. For example, our mind-body team routinely provides teaching to medical wards within the hospital and to schools (as part of discharge planning), and incorporates focus-of-attention into our general teaching about FND (including functional seizures). Some examples include the following:

> Having learnt pain management in the postoperative setting, a nurse new to the Mind-Body Program asked Zbigniew — a 13-year-old boy with functional seizures and functional abdominal pain — to assess his pain using a standard pain scale multiple times during her shift. The boy always reported significant pain, and in the period following the nurse's questioning, he was no longer able to enjoy the interactions with his roommate. He was also unable to eat; instead, he would start to clutch his stomach and groan. When, on the advice of the mind-body team, the nurse stopped asking about Zbigniew's pain, she was surprised that he did not report pain on her shift. She also noticed that his interactions with his roommate became more playful. In addition, Zbigniew did not show any observable behavioural signs of pain (groaning, clutching his stomach, refusing to eat).

> A public school employed a teacher's aide to facilitate the management of Jamie, an 11-year-old girl with functional seizures. The teacher's aide sat next to Jamie and watched out for the functional seizures — the aide saw her entire role as observing Jamie and being ready to notice her warning signs of a functional seizure. Although she never said this explicitly, all her body language communicated what she was doing. In contrast to Jamie's functioning in the hospital school — where the odd functional seizure had occurred — the number of seizures at the public school began to mount. After some education about attention and functional seizures, the mind-body team suggested that the teacher's aide be used as a class aide — so that her attention was not focused on Jamie. Within a few weeks the frequency of Jamie's functional seizures returned to the same low level as at the hospital school.

Setting Up Positive Expectations

In Chapter 8 we saw that the young person's expectations and the expectations of her family can have a powerful impact on shaping the treatment process and treatment outcomes. In this context it is the clinician's task — and the task of the multidisciplinary team as a whole — to set up positive expectations, in an ongoing way, in conversations with the young person and family.

During the Neurology (Medical) Assessment

The positive expectations that are set up by a well-conducted neurological assessment of functional seizures have the effect of propelling the therapeutic process in the right direction from the outset. The neurologist sets up positive expectations by the following: establishing a good therapeutic alliance; making a positive diagnosis of functional seizures (or FND if the functional seizures are comorbid with other functional neurological symptoms); providing a clear explanation (including the availability of successful treatment interventions) (Vassilopoulos et al., 2022); and directing the young person onto the appropriate outpatient or inpatient treatment pathway.

During the Biopsychosocial Assessment

In the biopsychosocial assessment, you, the clinician, can reaffirm the positive expectations that have been set up during the neurology (medical) assessment. Invariably, the young person and family will ask you many questions. They will want to know, among other things, what treatment entails, whether it is generally successful, and what percentage of young people regain health and wellbeing. Because clinical outcomes from programs for functional seizures in children and adolescents are very positive — 63% to 95% show full resolution of FND symptoms (Vassilopoulos et al., 2022) — you can cite the evidence, and you can underline that young people who engage in biopsychosocial treatment, with the support of their families, do well.

The following vignette shows the powerful nature of expectations in the process of recovery.

> Bernadette, an adolescent girl with an eight-month history of FND (including functional seizures) had missed out on admission to the Mind-Body Program because the program had been shut down during that particular period in the COVID-19 pandemic. She knew, however, that many young people made a full recovery by the end of the program's two-week inpatient hospital stay. When the program reopened, the girl was enthusiastic about her admission and engaged in every aspect of the program. She was particularly excited by her newly acquired mastery pertaining to focus-of-attention that is part of the Five-Step Plan (see section above). Because of this achievement, by the discharge date she was able to avert most of her functional seizures.
>
> The parents of Charles, a 12-year-old boy with functional seizures, were frustrated and angered by the unhelpful interactions that they had experienced in their journey through the medical system. At the assessment they felt hopeless about any improvement and kept referring to Charles as having a 'disability'. Moreover, they asked the

team about what renovations they would need to make to the home to support Charles in his lifelong illness. When the mind-body team reassured them that the team treated functional seizures all the time and that the treatment was effective in the majority of cases, Charles's parents were able to put aside their feelings and support Charles in accepting admission into the program. They shifted their frame for thinking about Charles and his medical situation: instead of his having a chronic, untreatable condition, he had a treatable condition from which, via the intensive work involved in the Mind-Body Program, he would recover. With the help of his parents, Charles was able to engage in all treatment components. On discharge home, Charles and his parents were confident that they could carry through the program. Charles was sad to leave the new friends he had made in the hospital school. Six weeks later Charles's functional seizures had settled.

To Frame the Treatment Process

We often use visual metaphors to depict the treatment process for the young person and the family (see Figure 9.1). For other metaphors — the staircase metaphor and path on a mountain metaphor — see Chapter 16 of Kozlowska, Scher, and Helgeland (2020).

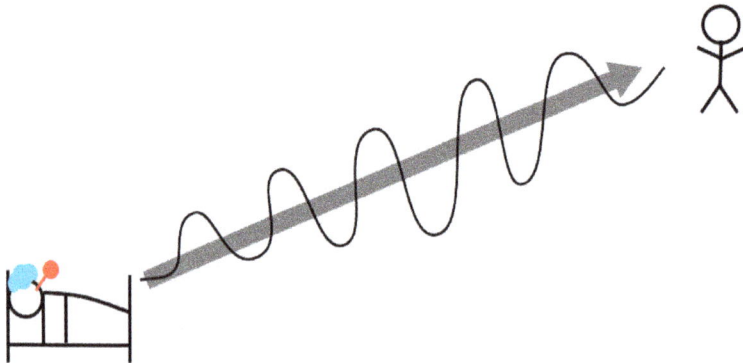

Figure 9.1 Wavy-line metaphor of the recovery process. The wavy-line metaphor depicts the ups and downs that are part of the recovery process. This metaphor can be drawn on a piece of paper, or it can be communicated nonverbally via hand gestures whilst the clinician is explaining the recovery process with the family. The thick, straight line represents the overall direction of the recovery process, which happens slowly over time. The wavy line represents the ups and downs that occur along the way. The clinician needs to emphasise the importance of maintaining hope and positive expectations, even when the young person, family, and treatment team find themselves in one of the troughs; the overall direction of change is toward health and wellbeing.
© Kasia Kozlowska 2022

During the Daily Process of Treatment

The treatment process may be very straightforward, or it may be long and difficult. In either scenario, the therapeutic task of maintaining hope and positive expectations needs to be integrated into all conversations and interactions in an ongoing way. In your conversations with the young person, you, the clinician, can use words, metaphors, and suggestions to illuminate a path forward, hoping to steer the young person toward healthy actions and healthy future outcomes (Erickson, 1954; Haley, 1973; Stoddard et al., 2014; Sugarman et al., 2020).[3]

Below are some simple examples of health-promoting suggestions embedded in our daily conversations with the young person.

'Wow, you were able to catch one of the warning signs! What a breakthrough! As you practise more and more, your skill will get better and better, better and better. It will be so interesting to see how you are doing on all this, day by day, day by day.'

'Now that you are sleeping better, and your body and brain are getting proper rest, all those renewal processes that we talked about with your family will start to kick in.[4] I think you will now find it much easier to implement some of those regulation strategies you've been practising.'

'You managed to get your breathing rate down to five breaths per minute on the biofeedback device. That's very impressive . . . far better than many adults. Breathing is a powerful tool in preventing functional seizures. I wonder what would happen in physio if you did the breathing the moment you start to panic.'

'Even though you didn't enjoy it, you were able to get to school today. I am so proud of you. You stayed in the classroom even though you didn't feel like it and really fought that anxiety. Every time you go to school, you'll get stronger and stronger, and more and more able to control the anxiety. You are the boss of your body!'

'I know that you can be really stubborn [said with humour]. I wonder what will happen when you put your stubborn mind to the work of getting better?'

---

3 Sidney Rosen captured this idea of using suggestion to steer the patient's path in his 1991 book *My Voice Will Go with You: The Teaching Tales of Milton H. Erickson.*

4 For a summary of the renewal processes that occur during sleep, see Chapter 5 of Kozlowska, Scher, and Helgeland (2020).

'Everyone we work with finds at least one or two regulation strategies that they are able to use. It will be interesting to see which ones suit you.'

'With other young people that we've worked with who struggle to eat, we usually find that having a smoothie or Ensure helps retrain their stomach and makes it easier to eat. We can explore this together, and you'll find out which one is best for you.'

Using Hypnosis to Affirm Positive Expectations

The trance, or hypnotic, state involves a state of focused attention — on something that is important, or that is suggested by the hypnotherapist — with reduced peripheral awareness (Kohen & Kaiser, 2014). Young people who are able to enter a trance state in a formal way (e.g., during a hypnosis session) have an enhanced capacity to respond to positive suggestions, which often play a major role in the results obtained through hypnosis. The sessions may include relaxation scripts and also scripts used for pain management (or for other purposes). Such scripts can be used, separate from any formal hypnosis session, by those unable to enter a trance state. Some of the young people that we have worked with have asked a parent to play to them, via ear plugs, the recorded version of a hypnosis session (with its embedded suggestions) when they are experiencing a functional seizure. These recordings help the young person to ride out the seizure (step 4 of the Five-Step Plan) and to reduce the time of the functional seizure.

Below we provide some examples of suggestions that we have used when the young person has been in a formal trance state during a hypnosis session or during a physiotherapy session (one undertaken with the young person in a trance state).

'When you come out of trance, you will carry these feelings of comfort with you for the rest of the day. And you will be able to enter this state of calm and relaxation whenever you would like to do so.'

'Because of your ability to use trance and hypnosis, you will be able to use the power of your mind to help your body settle when you notice the warning signs of a functional seizure.'

'Your body is like a tree moving in the wind or like grass swaying backward and forward in the breeze.' [suggestion of flexibility and movement introduced to a boy who suffered from symptoms of dystonia (which immobilised certain body parts into an unhealthy position)]

'Think of that picture of your nervous system [Figure 4.3]. Imagine your nervous system slowly switching off from red to blue and the feelings of calm sweeping through your body.'

In this chapter we have mainly discussed the positive suggestions that are part of ordinary conversation/therapy as separate from the positive suggestions that are part of formal hypnosis — when the young person is formally inducted into a trance state. It is important to note, however, that the processes are not that different. Contemporary hypnotherapists implement positive suggestion into their clinical encounters in a broader, more fluid way so that it becomes a pervasive part of the therapy process. For example, they might conceptualise that many patients — young and old — are already in a trance-like state in the clinical encounter and that a formal induction is not needed. They would simply proceed in utilising positive suggestion as part of every clinical encounter, with hypnosis, so conceived, as the cornerstone. Notably, this use of positive suggestion is not the sole 'property' of hypnotherapists. All health care professionals need to understand positive suggestion as one of the most useful skills in their professional toolbox.

For more information about contemporary conceptions of hypnosis (in particular, with young people), see Kohen and Kaiser's 2014 review of clinical hypnosis in children and adolescents, Helgeland and colleagues' 2022 article on clinical hypnosis, Helgeland's 2019 commentary on the case of Jai, for whom hypnosis was a vital part of the intervention for his difficult-to-treat functional neurological symptoms (Khachane et al., 2019), and Helgeland and colleagues' forthcoming chapter 'Hypnosis in the treatment of functional somatic symptoms in children and adolescents'. See also Chapter 10.

Working with the Mind III: Cognitive (Top-Down) Interventions and Regulation Approaches

In Chapter 8 we identified illness-promoting and illness-perpetuating psycho-logical processes, and in Chapter 9 we discussed two of these processes — focus-of-attention and expectations about the therapeutic process — in greater detail. In this chapter we discuss the introduction of top-down (cognitive) regulation strategies into the young person's skill set, along with a range of cognitive interventions that our mind-body team often utilises in our work with young people with functional seizures. Once the young person has mastered one or more cognitive regulation strategies, these strategies are integrated into steps 3 and 5 of the Five-Step Plan (see Chapter 6).

As noted earlier, visual representations of the Five-Step Plan are available in Appendix C (for the young person) and Appendix D (for the young person and parent [or other adult]). Both are suitable for printing, and translations of Appendixes C and D into some other languages are available online from the publisher.

Introducing Cognitive (Top-Down) Regulation Strategies into the Young Person's Skill Set

It is helpful for the young person to trial different cognitive strategies in therapy sessions. Once the young person has identified the most-liked strategies, you need to encourage her[1] to practise them four times a day for five minutes until she has mastered them. The young person can also try to implement them, alongside the neurophysiological (bottom-up) regulation strategies, when she

---

1 As noted in earlier chapters, because functional somatic symptoms occur more frequently in girls than in boys, we generally use the pronouns she and her to reflect this clinical reality.

notices her body becoming activated (aroused) or when she notices an unhelpful cognitive process occurring (e.g., she catches herself catastrophising). The practice of cognitive regulation strategies should be added to the young person's daily timetable (see Figure 10.2 later in this chapter).

The skill set that you, the clinician, bring to this component of the intervention — working with the mind — will depend on your training. If you have trained in a body-based tradition — somatic experiencing, sensory-motor therapy, and so on — you will already be skilled at helping the young person put aside her thought processes and shift her focus-of-attention to tracking body state. You will be less familiar, however, with working with cognitive processes per se. If you have training in second-wave cognitive-behavioural therapy (CBT) (Hayes & Hofmann, 2017), you will be very familiar with managing maladaptive thoughts — and you can utilise your entire skill set in this area — but you may be less familiar with working with focus-of-attention when attention is being pulled toward, and captured by, body-arousal sensations (see Text Box 10.1).

Text Box 10.1
The Three Waves of Cognitive-Behavioural Therapy

There have been three distinct waves of cognitive-behavioural therapy (CBT), with each wave reflecting 'dominant assumptions, methods, and goals' (Hayes, 2004, p. 640; Brown, 2011; Hayes, 2018).

Wave 1. *Behavioural* therapy was based on the work of Ivan Pavlov, Burrhus Frederic Skinner, and John Watson. It focused on observing, predicting, and modifying behaviour to promote change.

Wave 2. *Cognitive-behavioural* therapy, based on the work of Albert Ellis and Aaron Beck, focused on the link between dysfunctional cognitions and maladaptive behaviours. The objective was to alter these existing maladaptive patterns and to develop more adaptive ones.

Wave 3. The third wave of CBT integrates *mindfulness* strategies brought into Western practice by Jon Kabat-Zinn (1990, 2003, 2005), who studied Buddhist mindfulness teaching. The objective in mindfulness-based therapies (as integrated into third-wave CBT) is to help the young person to learn to live with painful or unpleasant sensations and with pain in the world, and to accept the way things are — instead of suffering by trying to change them. Third-wave CBT involves a diverse range of interventions, including Acceptance and Commitment Therapy, Mindfulness-Based Cognitive Therapy (MBCT), Trauma-Focused CBT, and Dialectical Behaviour Therapy (DBT). Many of these interventions use top-down, mindfulness-based, emotion-regulation strategies where the young person utilises intentional efforts to increase her attention and awareness capacities for better control of thoughts and feelings (Guendelman, 2017).

Contemporary CBT practitioners will usually integrate strategies from all three waves into their practice.

Adapted from Kozlowska, Scher, and Helgeland (2020) and Vassilopoulos and colleagues (2022).

The point we want to make is that as a mental health clinician, your training and your skill set already provide you with a significant part of the toolkit needed to work with young people with functional seizures. But you need to examine your toolkit carefully, pick out the elements that will help you with this patient group, and identify the elements that are missing — so that you can add them to your existing toolkit. This process may also require some relearning. For example, if you were trained in the era where CBT trainers taught that slow-paced breathing was a safety behaviour — a behaviour that reduced short-term anxiety but prevented longer-term cognitive change (Gelder, 1997; Thwaites & Freeston, 2005) — then you will need to replace this learning with a more contemporary understanding. Slow-paced breathing up-regulates the restorative parasympathetic system — calming the brain and body. In this way, slow-paced breathing may allow the young person to calm down sufficiently to bring the frontal lobe *online*, enabling her to utilise cognitive processes to regulate. When the frontal lobe is under stress, cognitive processes are difficult to utilise. In states of high arousal, reflexive motor-sensory processes — coupled with threat-related cognitions — are prioritised, and rational thinking is difficult (Arnsten, 2009, 2015).

Examples of Cognitive (Top-Down) Regulation Interventions and Strategies

In this section we discuss a handful of examples of cognitive regulation interventions and strategies that our mind-body team has found to be particularly useful in our work with young people with functional seizures.

Using the Sequencing Tool to Understand the Role of Cognitions

In Chapter 6 we used sequencing to help the young person identify the warning signs — the changes in body state — that marked activation of the body and that heralded the emergence of a functional seizure. In this component of the intervention — working with the mind — we use sequencing to identify how illness-promoting cognitions may play a role in activating the body prior to a functional seizure and how cognitions also play a role in activating the body at other times. In the sequence identified by Evie (below), we can see that the sequence of body sensations — marking a state of increased activation — was accompanied by illness-promoting thoughts that helped the activation process along (see Figure 10.1 and also Chapter 6).

The beauty of sequencing is that it allows you and the young person to depict the specific role of illness-promoting cognitions — as relevant to that particular young person — in visual form. The next step in the process is to identify strategies that the young person can practise — and that the family can help to implement — to disrupt the identified sequence.

```
┌─────────────────────────────────────┐
│  Feeling hot on the outside and cold │
│            on the inside             │
└─────────────────────────────────────┘
                  ▼
┌─────────────────────────────────────┐
│  Thinking 'this isn't normal', 'I'm  │
│        just going to ignore it'      │
└─────────────────────────────────────┘
                  ▼
┌─────────────────────────────────────┐
│  Having tension in the throat (a     │
│  globus sensation) and an unusual    │
│           taste in her mouth         │
└─────────────────────────────────────┘
                  ▼
┌─────────────────────────────────────┐
│           Breathing faster           │
└─────────────────────────────────────┘
                  ▼
┌─────────────────────────────────────┐
│  Having blurred vision and tingling  │
│           in the left arm            │
└─────────────────────────────────────┘
                  ▼
┌─────────────────────────────────────┐
│  Thinking 'I am going to push this   │
│  away', then trying to block out any │
│        of her bodily sensations      │
└─────────────────────────────────────┘
                  ▼
┌─────────────────────────────────────┐
│        Sharp pain in the chest       │
└─────────────────────────────────────┘
                  ▼
┌─────────────────────────────────────┐
│  Thinking 'here we go again', 'there's│
│  nothing I can do' 'this is out of my│
│  control'; feeling helpless and      │
│              hopeless                │
└─────────────────────────────────────┘
                  ▼
┌─────────────────────────────────────┐
│     Experiencing a functional        │
│             seizure                  │
└─────────────────────────────────────┘
```

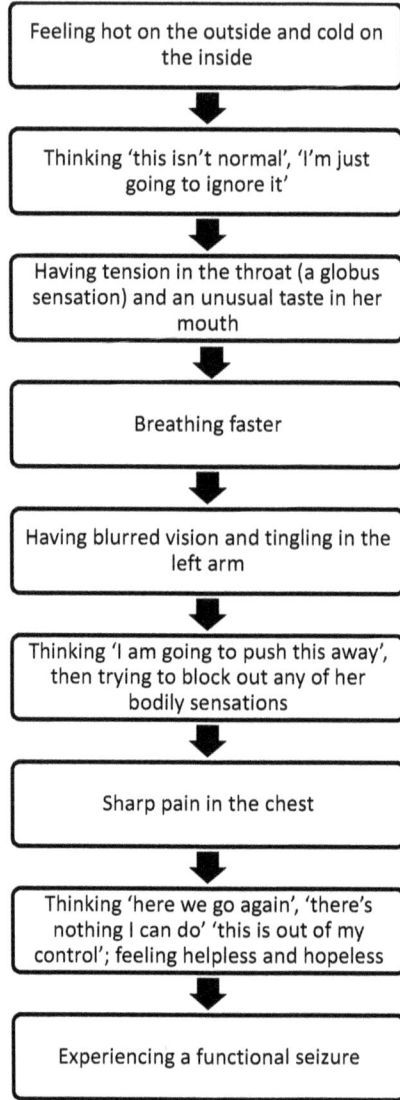

Figure 10.1 Evie's flowchart of warning signs and accompanying thoughts. This flowchart documents the final visual presentation of the sequence of events that preceded Evie's functional seizures: changes in body state (warning signs) and accompanying thoughts and feelings. © Kasia Kozlowska and Blanche Savage 2022

Managing Focus-of-Attention to Avert a Functional Seizure

As discussed in detail in Chapter 9, most young people with functional seizures require significant coaching and support to become adept at shifting attention as part of the Five-Step Plan. For completeness, in Text Box 10.2 we highlight

---

Text Box 10.2
Managing Focus-of-Attention During the Five-Step Plan

Step 1: Focus-of-attention on the felt sense of the body, the warning signs of the functional seizure
The young person needs to notice the felt sense of her body, moving her focus-of-attention to body sensations, the warning signs that a functional seizure is about to happen.

Step 2: Focus-of-attention onto the task of getting into a safe position
The young person needs to shift her focus-of-attention to the behavioural process of getting into a safe position on the ground to avoid falls and injury. In other words, as soon as she has recognized her warning signs (of an impending functional seizure), she needs to immediately shift her attention away from the warning signs and to the task to getting herself safe on the ground.

Step 3: Focus-of-attention on the regulation strategy
As soon as she is in a safe position, the young person needs to shift her focus-of-attention to the process of implementing a regulation strategy — either a neurophysiological (bottom-up) regulation strategy or a cognitive (top-down) regulation strategy.

Step 4: Focus-of-attention on riding it out
If the functional seizure is not averted, the young person needs to shift her focus-of-attention to the task of *riding it out.* The young person can either practise attending to her body sensations — even though they are unpleasant — with a curious, open stance (bottom-up mindfulness) or, if that is too difficult, focus on a self-affirming cognition (cognitive regulation strategy) such as 'OK, I can do it. It is not dangerous. It will not harm me. I have done it before. I am safe.'

Step 5: Focus-of-attention on the regulation strategy
As soon as the functional seizure is over, the young person needs to shift her focus-of-attention to the process of implementing a regulation strategy to further calm her body and brain (to a state of calm wellbeing).

© Kasia Kozlowska and Blanche Savage 2022

---

the manner in which the young person needs to manage focus-of-attention at each step of the Five-Step Plan.

Distraction

Distraction techniques involve any physical or mental activity that encourages the young person to redirect her focus-of-attention away from her activating body state and associated illness-promoting cognitions, to an external stimulus or activity. Common distraction techniques include things such as listening to music, drawing, talking to a parent, or reading a book. Because distraction is easy to implement, our mind-body team frequently uses it early on in step 3 of the Five-Step Plan. As the young person becomes more adept at a range of regulation strategies, distraction can be replaced by other bottom-up (see Chapter 7) and top-down (this chapter) regulation strategies.

Guided Imagery or Visualisation-Based Relaxation

Guided imagery and visualisation exercises have a long tradition in Western psychology (starting with psychodrama) and medicine (beginning with pain management in the treatment of cancer) (Academy for Guided Imagery, 1988–2022). Their use in Eastern healing traditions is presumed to be much longer. *Guided imagery* supports the young person in using her imagination — images (picture thoughts) that arise from the young person's own mind — to induce a calm body state that enables the young person to manage her distress and to down-regulate her arousal. By contrast, *visualisation* is used to prompt the young person's imagination through scripted images that are read aloud by the therapist. In current practice, most clinicians use these terms interchangeably.

The most common imagery that our mind-body team uses with the young person with functional seizures are scripts read by the clinician in which the young person imagines herself in a relaxing environment (e.g., on a rainforest walk or at the beach). The young person and therapist will discuss ahead of time which sort of setting she will find relaxing. These sessions are typically recorded on the young person's phone so that she can listen to recordings at set times during the day. For young people who prefer less-structured imagery, the clinician will coach them through the exercise of imagining that they are in a safe place (typically using all of their senses to enhance the experience of the place). Many resources are available online for therapists who are unsure where to start with guided imagery or visualisation. The safe-place exercise or other imagery-related exercises can be implemented as part of the young person's timetable (to calm her on a daily basis; see Figure 10.2 later in this chapter). They can also be used as the regulation strategy in step 3 of the Five-Step Plan, potentially averting a functional seizure (see Text Box 10.2 and also Chapter 6).

Because some young people's functional seizures are triggered by pain, imagery exercises designed to manage pain can be helpful in those particular cases. Such exercises involve strategies such as the following: to use colours to represent the pain in the body, and then practising changing the colour of the pain, shifting it to a preferred colour that is the opposite of the pain (e.g., diluting a red to a purple to a blue); to imagine shifting the pain colour out of the body (e.g., with every breath, imagine filling a balloon with the pain (colour) and then letting the balloon float up into the sky); or to imagine shifting one's awareness out of the body (e.g., to allow the mind to float freely away from the body and the pain). The last of these interventions is somewhat risky for some young people who may have a tendency to shift into an altered state (including a functional seizure). For this very reason, the interventions are initially practised in session with the therapist to see which are helpful and which are not.

Challenging Unhelpful Thoughts

As we saw in Chapter 8, during therapy with young people experiencing functional seizures, some of the most common themes — thoughts, feelings, and mental images — identified include the following:

- Helplessness: for example, 'There is nothing I can do about my seizures.'

- Hopelessness: for example, 'Nothing is ever going to change. I will be like this forever.'

- Catastrophising: for example, 'This is the worst thing that can happen to me. I am never going to be able to do anything I like.'

- Social worries: for example, 'I look like an idiot.'

- Black-and-white thinking: for example, 'If I have one seizure, it is all over. I am going backward. I have lost all my progress.'

In any of these scenarios, the second-wave CBT intervention of challenging or replacing unhelpful thoughts can be useful (Beck, 1976; Rapee et al., 2008).

> A boy who experienced a pounding heart as a warning sign before he had a functional seizure initially thought, 'My heart is pounding. There must be something physically wrong with me. I might be really sick.' His therapist helped him challenge these thoughts and replace them with 'It's just an anxious feeling . . . It won't hurt me.'

Exposure Coupled with the Implementation of a Neurophysiological Regulation Strategy and a Positive Cognition

This intervention draws from three different schools of psychotherapy: behavioural therapy (exposure), body-oriented psychotherapy (neurophysiological regulation), and second-wave CBT (helpful cognition that challenges the unhelpful cognition). Because they fear triggering another seizure, many young people with functional seizures avoid unpleasant body sensations and also situations that activate such sensations. This avoidance is unhelpful because it establishes a vicious cycle: the young person does less and less; the young person loses her sense of mastery and becomes more and more deconditioned; and the functional seizures increase in frequency.

In this exposure intervention the young person practises opening herself to experience the unpleasant situation or sensation and habituates to that experience. She practises this over and over again. During the exposure she can use body-based strategies (e.g., slow-paced breathing or progressive muscle relaxation) coupled with helpful cognitions (e.g., 'I can do this' or 'I can fight this') to help her stay in the situation long enough to habituate her anxiety.

Exposure Coupled with Sitting with, Tracking, and Tolerating Difficult Body Sensations

This intervention also involves opening oneself to experience difficult or unpleasant body sensations. It draws from two different schools of psychotherapy: behavioural therapy (exposure) and body-oriented psychotherapy (sitting with, tracking, and tolerating difficult body sensations). Because third-wave CBT — for example, Acceptance and Commitment Therapy (ACT) — has incorporated meditative techniques, some clinicians trained in ACT may be familiar with the idea of sitting with and tracking body sensations (a type of bottom-up mindfulness).

> Misha, a 12-year-old girl, struggled to identify any of her feelings or body states. This made it very challenging for her to notice her warning signs (step 1 of the Five-Step Plan). Misha and her therapist began with *easier* feelings — that is, those that were more acceptable to Misha. For example, the therapist asked Misha about the last time she had felt happy. Misha was able to identify a recent birthday party. She and the therapist then tracked back through the party in Misha's imagination, identifying what was happening, what she was feeling, where she noticed this feeling in her body, and what her body was doing at the time. Misha struggled with this exercise as it felt uncomfortable and unnatural to her. She kept wanting to rush through to the end of the party. The therapist had to keep bringing her back to the task and then keep moving through it very slowly. Misha and the therapist then engaged in a similar process — in imagination — again and again with different feelings. Eventually, Misha was able to track body states, including warning signs of her functional seizures, in the moment.

Sitting with Difficult Thoughts and Feelings

For young people who block out unpleasant feelings or thoughts, learning to sit with these can be difficult but helpful. This intervention borrows from the Eastern meditative traditions (and ACT in Western psychology) of accepting and allowing uncomfortable or unpleasant thoughts and feelings without struggling against them. It also uses some of the principles of habituation from behavioural therapy; that is, by sitting with an unpleasant thought or feeling, body arousal will decrease in unpleasantness with time.

Nadia was an 11-year-old girl presenting with onset of functional seizures following a medical procedure. During her individual therapy sessions, it became apparent that Nadia struggled to acknowledge and identify feelings of anger. This was partially due to religious beliefs: Nadia believed that feeling and expressing anger was unacceptable. The issue was discussed in that week's family session. Nadia's parents were then able to provide Nadia with alternative interpretations of the family's religious beliefs and were able to support Nadia to engage in the therapeutic work of learning how to identify and express anger. In sessions, Nadia and her therapist began to identify feelings that were adjacent to anger: irritation, frustration, annoyance. They practised noticing these feelings in the body and sitting with them. Once Nadia had mastered this skill, they began to notice and sit with more intense feeling states: anger, rage, and fury. To begin with, just talking hypothetically about anger — and feeling it just a little for a just a second — was confronting for Nadia. Gradually, she was able to sit with these feelings and the accompanying body sensations for a few minutes at a time. This section of the individual therapy took three months to complete.

Surfing the Wave: Riding Out the Functional Seizure

Sometimes the young person is unable to avert the functional seizure using her strategies. The surfing-the-wave strategy — riding out the functional seizure — is designed for these situations. The therapist prepares the young person for the eventuality that, to begin with, she will not be able to avert all of her functional seizures. Also, she needs to understand that once a functional seizure has taken hold, the best policy is to simply ride it out. In the Australian context, we use the analogy of surfing a wave because every child knows that once you have lost traction when surfing a wave, the best policy is to go with it — that is, to let the wave dump you and thrash you around, and then to swim back to the surface and begin all over again. This intervention is also similar to ACT strategies in which the young person does not *fight* the unpleasant sensation but lets it come and go. She chooses to allow the experience to be as it is, thereby strengthening her sense of mastery and self-agency.

Other Mindfulness Strategies

Mindfulness strategies come from Eastern traditions and have been incorporated into third-wave CBT. Mindfulness can be based on awareness of body sensations and therefore be part of neurophysiological interventions (bottom-up mindfulness as we have described in Chapter 7). It can also be a cognitive intervention, as when people practise awareness of their thoughts, feelings, or mental images (top-down mindfulness as described in this chapter).

Many resources are available online to help children and young people practise mindfulness. Our team recommends *Smiling Mind* to the young people we see, as it is a free app that is designed to be accessible for all ages.

Hypnosis

Clinicians trained in hypnosis can utilise their skills in formal hypnotic sessions but also informally in 'standard' clinical conversations (Helgeland et al., 2021). This informal use of hypnosis involves a natural, but careful, use of language that prioritises positive suggestion to promote health, mastery, and positive expectations in the young person (see Chapter 9). As such, the reader will recognise that this informal use of hypnosis is equivalent to what supportive therapists do with their patients, day in and day out.

Our mind-body team also uses formal hypnosis as a discrete regulation strategy that is implemented alongside other regulation strategies and alongside the informal use of hypnosis as described above — that is, the use of positive suggestion as an element of ongoing therapeutic conversations.

The formal use of hypnosis involves an initial assessment to determine whether the young person is able to achieve a trance state (formal hypnosis). Thereafter, in addition to working with the hypnotherapist in a trance state, the young person may be able to enter into a hypnotic trance through listening to recordings from the therapist, or she may learn how to reach a trance alone (self-hypnosis). For those who can enter a trance state, hypnosis can be used in the following ways:

- To achieve a state of relaxation and comfort
- To promote mastery, a subjective sense of inner strength, and enhanced awareness of inner resources
- To achieve a deep state of trance in which the young person can disconnect/step away from/separate from pain or from the angst caused by a current situation that is distressing her and activating her body
- For pain management (and to prevent functional seizures triggered by pain)
- To complete medical procedures or challenging physiotherapy interventions that trigger anxiety, pain, or functional seizures

For young people who are not able to achieve a trance state, guided imagery or visualisation-based relaxation can be used (see above).

For more information about hypnosis, see the references provided in Chapter 9.

Integrating Top-Down Regulation Strategies into the Timetable

Once the young person has some regulation strategies that she can use, she needs to practise them regularly throughout the day — with practice times integrated into the daily schedule (see Figure 10.2). These strategies can be layered with the bottom-up strategies that the young person learned in Chapter 7.

Therapeutic Options After the Functional Seizures Are Under Better Control

In this chapter — and in Chapters 6, 7, and 9 — we have focused on therapeutic interventions that our mind-body team uses to help the young person gain control of her functional seizures. But for many young people and their families, gaining control of the functional seizures is just the first step of the therapeutic process. Issues pertaining to unresolved loss or trauma, anxiety, depression, and self-harm, as well as difficulties with friendships or within the family, may all need to be addressed in a subsequent intervention. Such an intervention may require a referral to a well-established program (e.g., ACT or Dialectical Behaviour Therapy) or service (e.g., a mental health community centre or family therapy service), or to a private therapy clinic that offers trauma-focused work or longer-term psychotherapy. For a handful of young people — those who experience functional seizures in response to traumatic memories — the trauma-processing intervention may be central to gaining control over the functional seizures.[2]

---

2 See, for example, Ratnamohan and colleagues (2018).

7.00 am to 7.30 am	Wake up Practise slow breathing in bed before getting up Use my self-talk: 'I can get through the day. Just because I feel tired now doesn't mean it will be a bad day'
7.30 am to 8.00 am	Breakfast, get dressed, get ready for the day
8.00 am to 9.00 am	Leave for school Listen to playlist of 'happy music' in car on the way to school Tell myself "I can get through this"
9.00 am to 3.00 pm	School (Eat morning tea and lunch) Take stress ball & fidget toys into school to use in class
3.00 pm to 4.00 pm	Practise grounding strategies in car on the way home from school.
4.00 pm to 4.30 pm	Afternoon tea Practise slow breathing while listening to visualisation recording
4.30 pm to 5.00 pm	Half an hour of exercise with mum (walk the dog, jump on trampoline, or go for a swim)
5.00 pm to 6.00 pm	Homework (Monday, Tuesday, Wednesday) Gymnastics (Thursday) Youth Group (Friday)
6.00 pm to 7.30 pm	Free time
7.30 pm to 8.00 pm	Dinner Do 10-minute mindfulness exercise with dad after dinner
8.00 pm to 8.30 pm	Free time
8.30 pm to 9.30 pm	Start bedtime routine: Move phone out of room and log off any devices Have a cup of herbal tea Have a warm shower Practise slow breathing while listening to visualisation recording Read in bed
9:30 pm	Lights out and sleep

Figure 10.2 Timetable Integrating the Rhythms of Daily Living, Bottom-Up Regulation Strategies, and Top-Down Regulation Strategies

Chapter 11

Addressing and Treating Comorbid Mental Health Issues

The rate of comorbid mental health conditions in young people with functional seizures (and, more broadly, with functional neurological disorder [FND]) varies widely — from 22% to 80% of children and adolescents in different cohorts (Vassilopoulos et al., 2022). The most common comorbid mental health conditions are anxiety and depression. Anxiety or depression can emerge before the onset of the FND illness, during the FND illness, or after the FND illness has resolved. For some young people, their increased capacity to be aware of difficult thoughts, feelings, and experiences — a skill that is learnt during the treatment process — can unmask underlying anxiety and depression. Consequently, it is important for clinicians to assess for symptoms of anxiety and depression throughout the course of the mind-body treatment intervention.

To make things more complicated, illness-promoting psychological processes can be part of the young person's presentation — whether the young person meets diagnostic criteria for a mental health disorder or not (see Chapter 8). These processes play a fundamental role in activating the stress system and contributing to the processes that drive functional somatic symptoms (including functional seizures). They also function as a vulnerability factor for the development of anxiety, depression, and other mental health disorders (Beck, 1976; Hummel et al., 2021). In this context, it is important for clinicians to explore the broad range of psychological processes that may be contributing to the FND presentation and that increase the young person's risk of developing a comorbid mental health disorder or the risk of not recovering from a comorbid mental health disorder (see Chapter 8).

Common Challenges and Pitfalls

It is important to underline that not all young people with functional seizures have comorbid mental health issues. Likewise, not all young people with functional seizures have a history of emotional distress or emotional trauma. Sometimes functional seizures are triggered by physical stressors, with pain, a minor injury, or a viral illness being most common. In this context, clinicians need to keep an open mind — and open lens — when taking the young person's developmental history. Clinicians who conceptualise functional seizures as 'purely psychological' — or who doggedly probe for repressed trauma or emotional distress that is not present — are likely to elicit a negative response from the young person and her[1] family. Moreover, even when the clinician's beliefs are not explicitly articulated, the young person is likely to infer that the clinician thinks that the functional seizures are 'all in her head'. It is common, in any event, for this interaction to elicit feelings of distress and anger.

Another common difficulty in trying to assess for comorbid mental health conditions is that the young person may not resonate well with psychological constructs. For example, she may deny the subjective experience of depression. However, if you use a simple 0 to 10 Likert scale (see Figure 3.2), you may discover that her mood has dropped quite significantly. Or if you ask about the physical symptoms of depression — loss of energy, change in sleep patterns, and change in eating patterns — a different picture may emerge. As another example, the young person may not connect with the idea of panic attacks but may answer in the affirmative if you ask her about a pounding heart, feeling sweaty, butterflies in the stomach, nausea, or wanting to vomit — the physical symptoms of a panic attack. So, using language that resonates with the young person's experience is important. Language that captures the somatic narrative — the felt experience in the body — tends to resonate better than psychological constructs that evaluate experience on the cognitive system level — the level of thoughts and feelings.

Given these factors, you, the clinician, need to raise the idea of comorbid mental health conditions carefully and link them into a mind-body/biopsychosocial formulation (see Chapter 3). You should be giving the message that comorbid anxiety or depression often occurs alongside functional seizures — and other functional somatic symptoms — and that it can *contribute* to overactivation of the stress system (which is not to say that anxiety or depression, per se, caused the functional seizures). This information on comorbid disorders can then be

---

1 As noted in earlier chapters, because functional somatic symptoms occur more frequently in girls than in boys, we generally use the pronouns she and her to reflect this clinical reality.

included as one part of the biopsychosocial formulation that you develop with the family and young person (see Figure 11.1).

Treating Comorbid Mental Health Conditions

If the young person has a comorbid mental health condition, the following steps should be taken:

- The mental health condition should be discussed with the young person and her family. It should be put into the biopsychosocial formulation that you develop with the family (see Figure 11.1). The role of anxiety or depression in up-regulating or dysregulating the stress system should be discussed.

- Initiating treatment for the anxiety and depression as soon as feasible — whether with psychotherapy alone or in combination with medication — is important because resolution of comorbid mental health concerns is associated with better long-term outcomes (Kozlowska, Gray, et al., 2020). You will need to decide — depending on the young person's presentation and the extent of

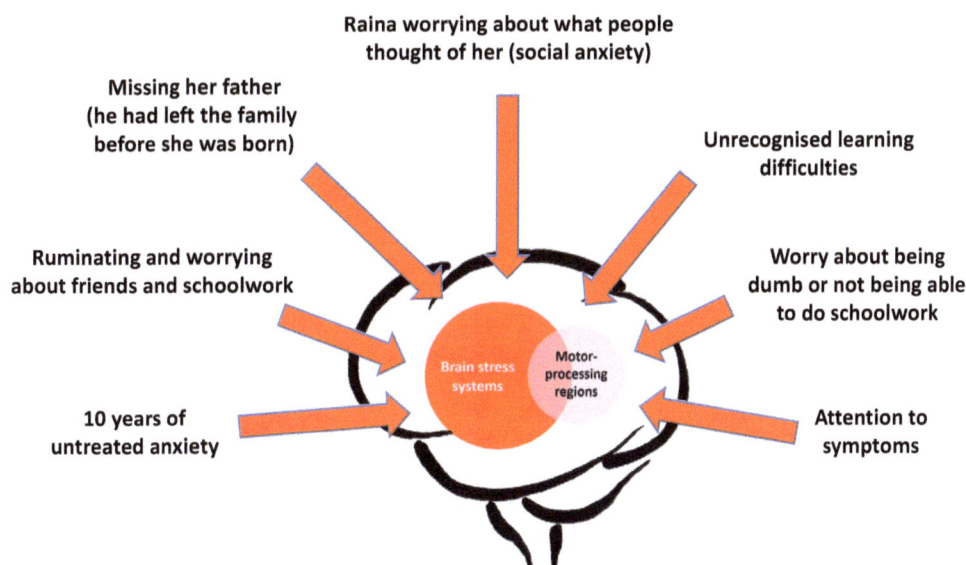

Figure 11.1 Raina's biopsychosocial formulation. A drawing of the formulation for a teenage girl (Raina). Raina's functional seizures presented against a background of significant untreated anxiety and unrecognised learning difficulties. In Chapter 11 we discuss Raina's case further to illustrate how our team supported Raina to return to school. © Kasia Kozlowska 2017

your own clinical resources — whether you provide this component of treatment concurrently with, or subsequent to, the intervention for the functional seizures (see Five-Step Plan in Chapter 6). In our Mind-Body Program, we generally initiate treatment for comorbid mental health problems as soon as possible, and then, when necessary, we provide referrals for ongoing management of these problems to a therapist or mental health team outside the program.

- Given that functional seizures indicate a high level of brain-body arousal — which the young person is struggling to regulate — it can be helpful to consider medication early in the treatment process (see Chapter 15 for further discussion of medications). This approach may differ from what you might do with a young person presenting only with anxiety or depression, where you would try psychotherapy first (e.g., CBT) and add medication only if subsequently needed. Untreated anxiety or depression will negatively affect the young person's capacity to manage her functional seizures (and other functional neurological symptoms), especially when the young person's illness is severe.

As in all therapeutic work with children, the treatment of anxiety and depression involves a social intervention where contributing factors in the family, school, and peer settings are addressed.

Chapter 12

Working with the Family

Working with the family is an integral part of the treatment program for young people with functional seizures. The family work should take place in parallel with the young person's individual work. The crucial importance of this family work, including the attendance of family members at therapy sessions, is best discussed with the family early on in the therapeutic process as part of their psychoeducation. Our mind-body team has found it helpful to meet with the *whole* family, including siblings and anyone else (such as a grandparent) living at home, at least once, typically at the biopsychosocial assessment session (see Chapter 3). This initial assessment promotes a holistic understanding of the child's symptoms as arising in the context of the child's — and family's — lived experience. It also promotes the ongoing involvement of the family in the therapeutic process.

Depending on the goals of subsequent family sessions, the sessions may be attended by the young person and both parents, by both parents alone, or by other combinations of individuals. It is usually unhelpful to meet with each parent separately unless there has been an acrimonious separation. In the latter case, the parents should be seen in separate sessions — with or without the young person (the primary concerns being the young person's safety and therapeutic progress). Our mind-body team has also found it helpful to use the term *family work* rather than *family therapy*. Whereas *all* families understand the need for the clinician(s) and family to work together as a collaborative team, *some* families do not see themselves as in need of family therapy.

Goals for Family Work: Teasing Apart Short-Term and Long-Term Goals

Overarching considerations in family work are that it be both directive and containing. Families with a young person who has presented with functional seizures are usually in a state of acute stress and distress due to their child's illness. Both short- and long-term goals need to be established. The former are shared by all families and the latter relate to the specific needs of each family.

Short-term goals typically include the following:

- Contain and support parental anxiety.

- Coach and support the parents in managing the functional seizures (as part of the Five-Step Plan; see Chapter 6).

- Teach the parents the mind-body regulation strategies that the young person is learning (so that they can support the young person in her[1] efforts).

- Explore, address, and contain any medical trauma (so that past adverse experiences do not disrupt the current therapeutic process).

- Assess for any relevant family issues that may be increasing stress in the home.

As noted earlier, visual representations of the Five-Step Plan are available in Appendix C (for the young person) and Appendix D (for the young person and parent [or other adult]). Both are suitable for printing, and translations of Appendixes C and D into some other languages are available online from the publisher.

Family issues that become identified as long-term goals of family work and that require a longer-term family intervention often become evident during the treatment program. It is helpful to make these issues explicit and to add them to the biopsychosocial formulation that was started with the family during the initial assessment (see Figure 12.1).

Common longer-term goals include the following:

- Addressing family *interactions* that contribute to stress levels at home. Common issues include parental conflict, unhelpful sibling interactions, problematic communication styles, and marital problems.

- Addressing family *processes* that contribute to stress levels at home. Common processes include the systematic failure to recognise or address strong emotions, with the consequence, for example, that grief or trauma (in individual or multiple family members) remains unaddressed and has a continuing negative effect on individual wellbeing and family dynamics. Sometimes the unresolved trauma relates to adverse experiences in the medical system.

---

1 As noted in earlier chapters, because functional somatic symptoms occur more frequently in girls than in boys, we generally use the pronouns she and her to reflect this clinical reality.

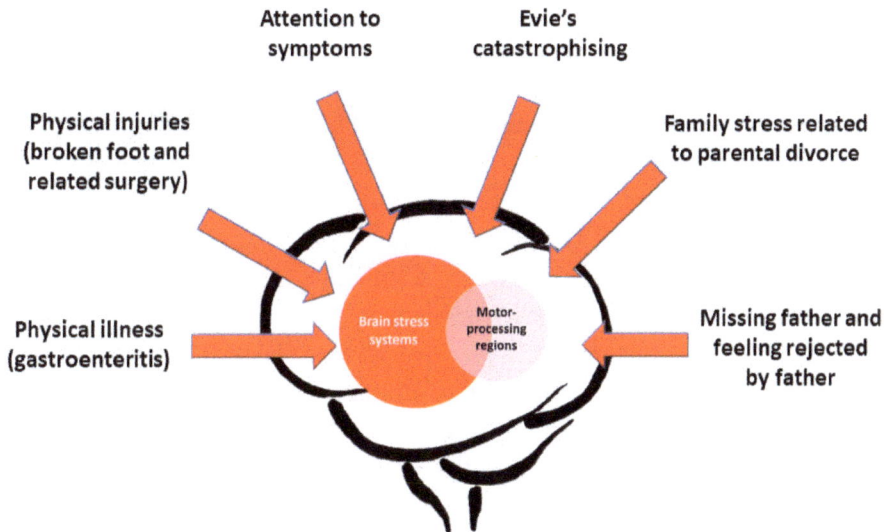

Figure 12.1 Evie's biopsychosocial formulation. A drawing of the formulation for a teenage girl (Evie). Evie's functional seizures presented against a background of significant family issues, which are included in the formulation. © Kasia Kozlowska 2017

- Addressing untreated health concerns — physical or emotional — within the family that contribute to the young person's worries and that play a role in maintaining activation of the young person's stress system.

The long-term goals may be addressed through a different therapeutic approach — for example, reflective family therapy — that is typically not as directive and containing as the initial work with the family. It is anticipated that the family's acute state of stress and distress will have settled by the time they start reflective family therapy. It is also anticipated that the young person's functional seizures will be improved and that the family now has the emotional space to focus more broadly on other issues that have been identified as contributing to the young person's presentation. In our Mind-Body Program, we are generally unable to provide reflective family therapy as part of our standard, two-week inpatient intervention, but we make referrals if reflective family therapy is indicated. Just how you proceed and what care is actually available to the family will depend upon the resources of your particular service (or another) within your institution or organisation, upon the professional resources in the community, and also upon the family's own financial resources.

In the sections below we discuss the therapeutic process pertaining to the short-term goals indicated above.

Containing Parental Anxiety

A number of structural interventions can be very effective in containing parental anxiety. These include the following: providing a clear biopsychosocial formulation (see Chapter 3), providing psychoeducation about functional seizures (see Chapter 4), having a clear treatment plan (see Chapter 3), scheduling regular parent sessions, and providing information about outcomes — namely, that most young people with functional seizures who engage in the treatment program will fully recover. Clinicians can also help to contain parental anxiety through their own nonverbal communication — that is, by staying calm, having a relaxed body posture, and not becoming defensive. What is thereby communicated nonverbally to the parents is how they can maintain a calm neurophysiological state — which is exactly what they need to do in order to calmly support their child in the Five-Step Plan (for details, see below).

Some clinicians may find it uncomfortable to abandon their typical stance in therapy — as one who asks open questions — and, with the parents, to take on the role of an *expert*. An important element of the expert role is to communicate an air of calm while confidently providing the parents with authoritative information that their child is safe, that she will learn how to manage her functional seizures, and that she will very likely return to a state of health and wellbeing. Notably, your capacity to take this stance and to communicate the information in question — both verbally and nonverbally — can be very containing for parents.

For some parents, however, the above interventions are insufficient to contain their anxiety about their child. If so, we recommend 'leaning in' to the parent's anxiety. Clinicians will often try to avoid anxious parents because these parents can eat up a lot of clinical time. Unfortunately, such avoidance usually has the effect of exacerbating the parents' anxiety. Instead, we suggest making more frequent contact with the parents — for example, having regularly scheduled phone calls in between face-to-face sessions — both to reduce their uncertainty and to communicate to them that they have a regular, designated time to raise any concerns or problems with you (see vignette of Ginny, below).

Coach Parents in How to Manage a Functional Seizure

The Five-Step Plan — or, for younger children, the Traffic Light Safety Plan — is outlined in Chapter 6.

The key components for parents are the following:

- It is ultimately going to be the young person's job to monitor and manage her body. As much as parents may want to, they cannot regulate their child's body for her. For many parents this learning point is difficult to process and accept; the task of stepping back and giving the child space to manage herself is extremely challenging. Achieving this component may require parents to engage in therapeutic work regarding their own anxiety, feelings, thoughts, self-expectations, and conceptions of themselves as good parents.

- Parents can help their child when she is having a functional seizure by staying calm and in control. If one parent finds it too distressing to be around the young person when she is having a functional seizure, the agreed plan may need to be for that parent to leave the room and for the other parent to stay.

- Parents can check that the young person is in a safe location when the functional seizure starts (e.g., is not likely to bang her head), but then the best approach is to minimise attention and to monitor the young person from a distance (i.e., in the same room, but not right next to the young person). Both by tone of voice and by behaviour, parents can communicate to the young person that they are not panicked and that everything will be okay. If parents can 'get on with things' and show that they are not worried, it will help the young person's nervous system calm down faster.

Figure 12.2 — which was first introduced in Chapter 6 — shows how these components are integrated into the Five-Step Plan for Managing Functional Seizures. The left-hand column shows the five steps that the young person needs to practise in order to learn, with time, to avert her functional seizures, and the right-hand column shows the five steps that the parent (or supervising adult) needs to practise in order to support the young person in her endeavour.

How the Coaching Process Looks in Real Life: A Vignette Example

Ginny, a teenage girl with a six-month history of acute anxiety and panic attacks — treated by an experienced clinician and clinical team at her local community mental health centre — began to experience functional seizures. The formulation of the mental health team was that anxious family interactions were maintaining the symptoms. For example, Ginny's parents demonstrated a range of anxiety-driven intrusive behaviours: not leaving their teenager alone, constantly asking how she was feeling, and not allowing her to do age-appropriate activities such as going out with friends. The mental health team treated this situation with a reflective family therapy intervention. The therapist reported, however, that therapy sessions were dominated by the parents' uncontained anxiety; they were both ruminating and catastrophising about what was going to happen to Ginny. The therapist reported that the anxiety was

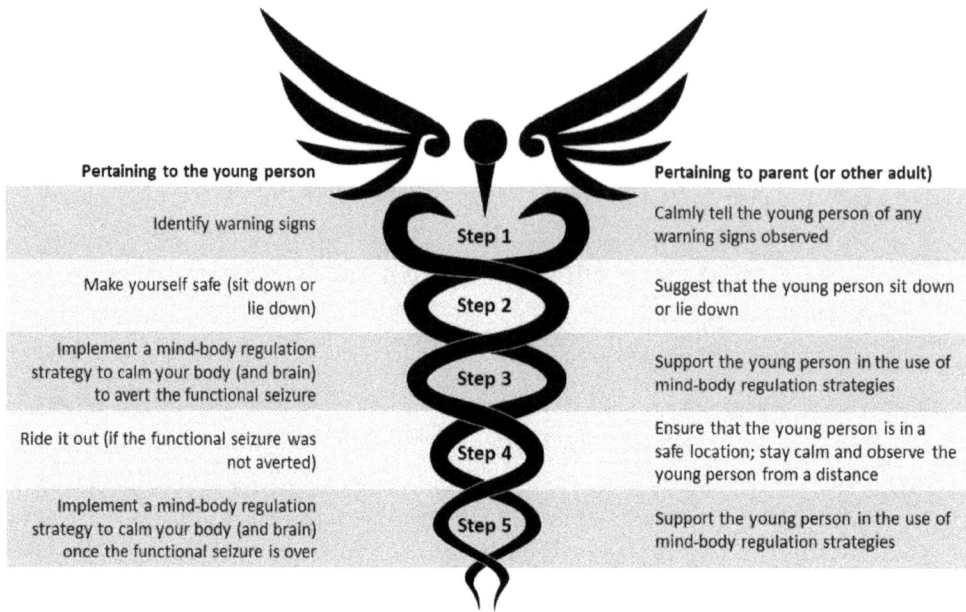

Pertaining to the young person		Pertaining to parent (or other adult)
Identify warning signs	Step 1	Calmly tell the young person of any warning signs observed
Make yourself safe (sit down or lie down)	Step 2	Suggest that the young person sit down or lie down
Implement a mind-body regulation strategy to calm your body (and brain) to avert the functional seizure	Step 3	Support the young person in the use of mind-body regulation strategies
Ride it out (if the functional seizure was not averted)	Step 4	Ensure that the young person is in a safe location; stay calm and observe the young person from a distance
Implement a mind-body regulation strategy to calm your body (and brain) once the functional seizure is over	Step 5	Support the young person in the use of mind-body regulation strategies

Figure 12.2 Five-Step Plan for Managing Functional Seizures (pertaining to the young person and the parent or supervising adult).
© Kasia Kozlowska and Blanche Savage 2022

so intense that she was actually struggling to contain her own neurophysiological state — and not just those of Ginny and her family. Because Ginny's functional seizures were worsening, and because of the clinician's request for help, Ginny was accepted into the hospital's Mind-Body Program.

Knowing that containment of anxiety was a primary therapeutic goal, our mind-body team set up a clear structural intervention with the family: visits with Ginny only at the set visiting times (to give her space), weekly family meetings with the mind-body team, and scheduled phone calls with the team twice a week. In the family sessions we took an *expert* stance and were very directive about what we wanted the parents to do — and not do — in their interactions with Ginny. When the parents struggled to follow our directions, our team supported them with their struggles and coached them to practise doing what they needed to do (see previous section). Slowly, the parent's anxiety settled, and Ginny's anxiety also started to settle.

During this therapeutic process, our team developed a good relationship with Ginny and her family. Once Ginny was on her way to recovery, the parents were able to compare and contrast their two experiences of therapy: the reflective family therapy with the community mental health team and the directive approach taken by our team. When talking about the former, Ginny's mother said:

> The therapist kept asking me how I would like to manage the situation . . . If I'd known what to do, I wouldn't have had to go to therapy! Whenever I asked the therapist what I should do, she wouldn't give me a clear answer.

Parents Who Struggle with the Five-Step Plan May Need Extra Coaching

Some parents struggle immensely to implement the Five-Step Plan. If this happens, they will need extra support in order to learn and master their five steps. You need to identify and then address, if possible, the barriers that are preventing the parents from following the plan. Common barriers include the following:

- Worry about their child being in pain or suffering

- Worry about 'abandoning' their child when their child needs them

- Concern about what other people might think of them for leaving their child to have a functional seizure

- An inability — despite their best intentions — to contain their anxiety and their worry about what might be happening to their child

- Overwhelming anxiety that overrides the parents' ability to think clearly in the moment and that activates autonomic, threat-related responses that they find difficult to modulate

- The triggering of the parents' own unresolved loss or trauma issues that may need to be addressed before they can fully support their child

These barriers can be addressed through thought challenging, psychoeducation, or coaching. Sometimes parents may need to learn and implement their own regulation strategies in order to be sufficiently calm and mindful that they can effectively support their child. When the clinician is very clear and concrete about what to do and what not to do, it can be very containing and can also, for some families, significantly decrease their ambient anxiety.

Sometimes parents will not be able to clearly identify or articulate the barriers preventing them from following the plan. In such situations, a bit of in vivo coaching might be effective, with you helping to support or coach the parents as they respond to an actual functional seizure.

Some parents may think that they are following the plan described above, but in fact they are paying attention to the functional seizures in subtle ways. Just what is happening may become apparent through unpacking in detail what the parent does when the young person has a functional seizure. Options include using a sequencing intervention (see Chapter 6) in which the temporal order of events is carefully mapped out with the parent, or observing the parent manage a functional seizure. Some of the subtle ways that parents may be drawing attention to a functional seizure include the following:

- Asking the young person 'How are you feeling?' or 'Do you think you might be about to have a functional seizure?'

- Nonverbal cues (such as the expression on the parent's face)

- Pressuring the young person to use her strategies and emoting disapproval if she does not

- Stroking the young person's hair during a functional seizure

- Supporting the young person's head during a functional seizure

- Videoing or recording the functional seizures (when doing so is no longer necessary because the diagnosis has been confirmed and the neurologist needs no further recordings; see Chapter 2)

Teach the Parents the Mind-Body Strategies That the Young Person Is Learning

Parents need to understand the rationale and techniques of the mind-body strategies that the young person is learning. When they do, parents are able to scaffold and coach the young person in using these strategies when appropriate. It also means that the parents themselves can use these strategies if needed.

This intervention can be implemented in joint parent-child sessions if their relationship is good enough to support the process. One way to do this is to have the young person teach the parents each strategy after she has learnt the strategy herself. The clinician can be present to ensure that the young person is giving an accurate description (or demonstration).

Resolving Iatrogenic Trauma

A small but significant portion of families with a young person presenting with functional seizures will previously have had negative experiences with the medical system (Kozlowska et al., 2021). These experiences can include misdi-agnosis, taking a long time to receive a diagnosis, having multiple unnecessary medical investigations, receiving an ambivalent diagnosis (e.g., 'It's not epilepsy'), being dismissed by medical staff ('Just ignore them and they'll go away'), being accused by medical staff of faking the functional seizures, and being denigrated by medical staff ('You're being hysterical'). Such adverse experiences are in and of themselves stressful, and they contribute to activation of the young person's stress system. These experiences can also put in jeopardy the engagement process because they arouse strong feelings of anger and resentment toward health care professionals. In this context it is important to address the young person and family's earlier adverse experiences within the medical system. These issues need to be addressed both explicitly and implicitly in your work with the family:

- Listen to the family's story. Allow them to tell the story of their child's illness and the medical investigations. Validate their perceptions and experience, and be sure that they understand that what happened shouldn't have happened.

- Be aware that adverse experiences in the medical setting can heighten a family's anxiety.

- Some families may need to access specific trauma-focused therapy in order to address any lasting impacts of their adverse experiences in the medical system.

- When needed, advocate for the young person and her family in the medical system. Advocate for them to be provided with a clear positive diagnosis. If the young person develops new or different functional somatic symptoms (not just a different type of functional seizure), advocate for these symptoms to be properly medically assessed and diagnosed.

Returning Back to Normal Function

In the same way that the return to normal function is a key goal for the young person with functional seizures, it is also a key goal for the young person's parents and family. In some cases, parents may need to be encouraged to return to work and reengage in the range of activities that were part of their lives before their child became ill with functional seizures. The family's return to normal function communicates a powerful message to the young person with functional seizures — namely, that all is well and that everyone's anxiety has now settled.

Chapter 13

Working with the School

The ultimate goal of the treatment program for functional seizures is for young persons to recover their normal capacity to engage in developmentally appropriate life activities. For most of these young persons, the goal will therefore be for them to return to school full time; it is consequently important for mental health clinicians (or the health care team) to work closely with the school. For older youth the goal may be for them to return to work or to their higher-education programs. More broadly, consolidating the connection to the school or work environment, along with eliminating or managing any barriers that can disrupt this connection, is important because these social aspects of life are central determinants of health and quality of life across the lifespan (Asadi-Pooya et al., 2021).

In our experience, many school staff find it helpful when we highlight that functional seizures are the product of *stress* and are even sometimes referred to as *stress-related seizures*. To remind the reader of this point, we often use the expression *functional (stress) seizures* in this chapter on working with the school. As we have stated elsewhere, functional seizures are a type of *functional neurological symptom disorder*, usually referred to, more simply, as *functional neurological disorder*, or FND.

We use the term *health care team* to refer to the set of health professionals who may, depending upon the setting and the needs of the young person and family, be involved in their clinical care. Also, because we are discussing the young person's return to school, we use the terms *young person* and *student* interchangeably.

From the perspective of the mental health clinician — or health care team — the key goals for working with the school include the following:

- Gathering collateral information from the school as part of the biopsychosocial assessment

- Including the school as a member of the young person's multidisciplinary team

- Providing psychoeducation to school staff — in this case, education about functional (stress) seizures

- Working with the school to develop a school-based health care plan for managing functional (stress) seizures in the school setting

- Organising an individualised, graded return to school (≈partial attendance) as a stepping stone to full-time attendance

- Working with the school to develop an individualised learning plan, or ILP (when needed)

- Identifying and implementing any needed special considerations (e.g., in taking exams) and obtaining, if available, any needed extra supports, including funding

- Problem-solving with the school — that is, working with school staff to address any barriers that could disrupt or complicate the young person's return to school

- Advocating for the young person and family, and promoting a good home–school relationship.

Gathering Collateral Information from the School as Part of the Biopsychosocial Assessment

The school is a rich source of information about the young person, the family, and their social circumstances. Speaking to the school is part of the biopsychosocial assessment. The goal of this conversation is to collect collateral information from the school regarding the young person's functioning: social functioning with peers, academic functioning, any specific attentional or learning difficulties, and any other issues that have come to the attention of the school. This potentially wide-ranging discussion has the additional advantage of enabling the health care team to engage with the school very early in the treatment — a vital step in bringing the school on board as part of the multidisciplinary team.

Including the School as Part of the Multidisciplinary Team

Attendance at school plays a key part in the young person's treatment and recovery, and is also an outcome goal of the treatment process itself. The school is therefore always a key member of the multidisciplinary team that provides coordinated care to the young person with functional (stress) seizures and that supports the young person's progress across the treatment process (see Figure 13.1). In the clinical experience of our hospital's mind-body team, if the school is not on board with this process, then the young person's recovery is adversely affected, and the health outcome is more likely to be poor. Fortunately, schools usually *are* on board. But sometimes the health care team has neglected to invite the school to be a collaborative member of the team, and sometimes the invitation comes too late. In yet other cases, the school, for one reason or another, does not position itself to cooperate.

Providing Psychoeducation

The discussion with the school needs to include psychoeducation about functional (stress) seizures. This education can include the information

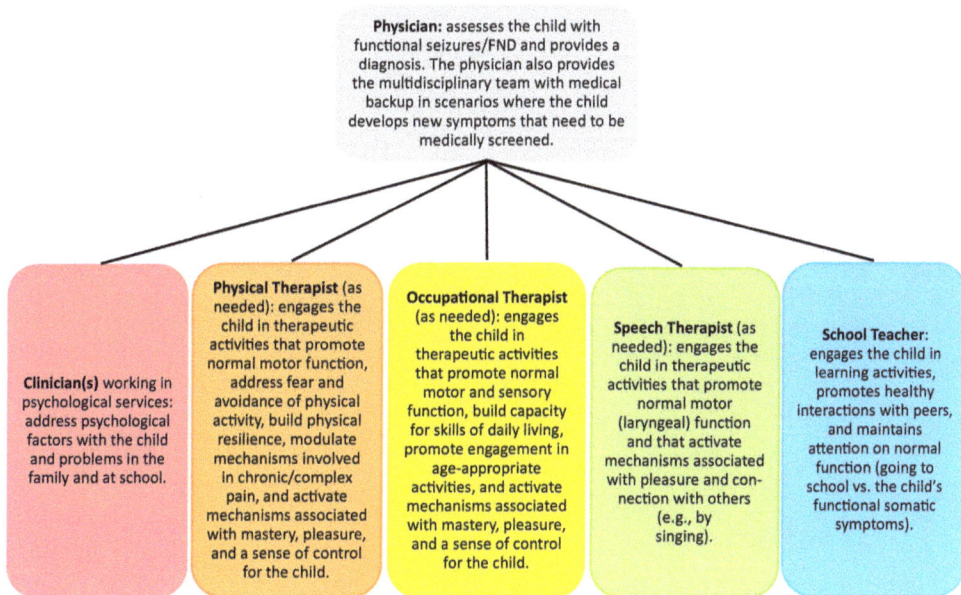

Figure 13.1 Multidisciplinary team. This figure represents the various professionals who may be part of the multidisciplinary team for a young person presenting with functional neurological disorder (including functional seizures). A physician, clinicians from psychological services, and staff from the young person's school are included on every team. A physiotherapist, occupational therapist, speech therapist, and other allied health professionals (e.g., art, music, and recreational therapists) join the team as required. ©Kasia Kozlowska 2021

previously provided to the family (see Chapter 4). Key points include the following:

- Functional (stress) seizures are a type of *functional neurological disorder* (FND). The student (and the family) may have been told that the student has 'FND with functional seizures' or just that the student has functional seizures. Other common names for functional seizures include *stress seizures, psychogenic non-epileptic seizures, dissociative seizures*, and *pseudoseizures* (see Figure 4.2). All these terms refer to the same thing. The terms most acceptable to young people are functional seizures, stress seizures, or non-epileptic seizures.

- Functional seizures need to be diagnosed by a paediatric neurologist or paediatrician. The diagnostic process involves a comprehensive medical examination (with appropriate investigations) that has confirmed that the student's events are functional — that is, stress related. The doctor has also confirmed that the events are not related to any other medical condition, such as epilepsy, low blood sugar in the context of diabetes, or a heart problem.

- Functional seizures can be very confronting when they are first witnessed in a school environment. They can be confronting for both staff members (who are expected, after appropriate training, to be able to manage functional seizures calmly) and for other students at the school. They are also distressing for the young persons themselves.

- Functional seizures reflect the stress-related overactivation of brain networks. In a nutshell, brain networks activate with stress. When the young person's brain networks activate too much and for too long, normal brain function is disrupted, and a functional (stress) seizure may result.

- The stress experienced by the student may involve one big event or lots of little stressors over time. Common stressors in the school setting include the following: starting a new school, difficulties managing academic pressures or expectations, undiagnosed learning difficulties, effects of anxiety on learning capacity, problems with friends, social exclusion, and teasing or bullying. A combination of stressors is often seen. Common physical stressors include pain, pushing too hard at sports, fatigue, hyperventilation, a minor injury, a viral illness, or a medical procedure. Common psychological stressors include worry about a family member and conflict in the family setting.

- When students experience functional seizures, they lose control of their bodies and may experience abnormal movements, loss of body tone, difficulty thinking clearly, and sometimes a change or even loss of consciousness.

- Functional seizures are different from epileptic seizures. Epileptic seizures are caused by sudden, abnormal electrical discharges in the brain. Functional seizures can look just like epileptic seizures (to the lay observer), but they are not caused by abnormal electrical discharges. Instead, they are triggered by stress and states of high arousal.

- It is common for functional seizures to change in the way that they present over time, whereas epileptic seizures are typically very stereotyped — fixed in their pattern of presentation for any particular person. An analogy is that functional seizures are like a chameleon that keeps changing colour, whereas epileptic seizures are like normal lizards, which always look the same.

- Functional seizures are not dangerous in themselves — they do not cause any injury to the young person's brain — though students need to learn to protect themselves from falling when functional seizures occur.

- Students with functional seizures have a very good prognosis if they engage in appropriate treatment. Outcome studies show that the majority of young persons who engage in treatment programs recover from functional seizures (Vassilopoulos et al., 2022). The prognosis for adults with functional seizures is generally less good, which reinforces the importance of treating functional seizures early and aggressively.

Our hospital's mind-body team has found it helpful to provide the school with a handout about functional seizures — one that can be distributed to all school staff involved in the student's care. Appendix B is a fact sheet about functional seizures suitable for printing and distribution; translations of Appendix B into some other languages are available online from the publisher. For further information see Appendix B.

School-Based Health Care Plan for Managing Functional Seizures

As noted above and in Chapter 2, the diagnosis of functional seizures is typically made by a paediatric neurologist or paediatrician. Once established, the health care team needs to provide the school, in a timely manner, a health care plan for managing the student's functional seizures if they occur at school. This *school-based health care plan*[1] should follow the principle of 'coordinated support' whereby the clinical team provides the school with the plan itself, with the school determining, in turn, how to best implement the plan in its particular educational setting. A simple, well-defined, school-based health care plan in written form is the most effective way of facilitating the school's efforts.

Key points pertaining to the management of functional seizures in the school setting are as follows:

- Functional seizures are not dangerous: they do not cause any injury to the young person's brain. There is no need to phone for an ambulance if a student has a functional seizure at school.

- If students notice their warning signs of a functional seizure when at school, they should — immediately — sit themselves down on the ground and implement their regulation strategies in an effort to down-regulate their arousal (calm down) and avert the functional seizure (see Five-Step Plan in Chapter 6). This step of the intervention is of the greatest importance because it helps prevent falls and injuries, and ensures that the student is able to stay safe in the school setting.

- When students have a functional seizure at school, only one adult is needed to monitor the situation, and this adult can do so from a distance. The rest of the class should continue with their work as usual. In the primary school setting, it can be helpful to have a bean bag available in the corner of the room, enabling students to retreat and to engage in their regulation strategies — to 'ride out' their functional seizures (see Five-Step Plan in Chapter 6).

- After having a functional seizure, students may need to go to the sick bay, library, or other available room for 15–20 minutes to use their regulation strategies to calm down (unless otherwise specified in their school-based health care plans; see Figure 13.2 and Five-Step Plan in Chapter 6)). Following this break, they can return to their usual activities.

---

1 In this manual we use the term *school-based health care plan* because it is self-explanatory. We are aware, however, that many different terminologies are used in different jurisdictions within Australia and around the world.

- The student should be able to participate in all school activities, including sport. Exceptions include swimming, abseiling, rock climbing, and other activities where the risk of injury — in the case of a functional seizure — may be difficult to manage.

To Whom It May Concern:

Re Kate Jones

DOB 28.11.2009

Kate is a patient at the Local Community Mental Health Team for treatment of functional seizures.

Kate experiences functional seizures, which are the body's way of responding to anxiety and stress. These are not epileptic seizures and are not dangerous. Kate has been fully investigated by a paediatric neurologist and her symptoms are not due to a medical cause (i.e., her seizures are not epileptic, nor are they caused by diabetes, low sugar level, or other medical causes).

The treatment for functional seizures is to manage stress in the body whilst returning to normal functioning. During her treatment with our team, Kate has learnt to identify early warning signs for her episodes and been taught strategies to bring her body's arousal down including slow breathing, visualisation and using fidget toys.

As part of Kate's treatment, she should return to school. To assist with Kate's return to school, the following management plan is recommended for her functional seizures.

MANAGEMENT PLAN FOR FUNCTIONAL SEIZURES

- Kate's episodes are not epileptic seizures and are not dangerous. There is no need to phone an ambulance or apply first aid unless her episode has caused other injuries.
- When Kate notices her early warning signs, she is to get to a safe place (on the ground) and use her strategies of slow breathing, visualisation (Kate has a recording on her phone she can listen to), and fidget toys.
- Kate's warning signs that she is about to have a functional seizure include dizziness, chest pain, and tingling in her fingers.
- If Kate has a functional seizure, there is no need to intervene except to ensure that she is safe (e.g., that she will not hit her head) and wait for the episode to pass. One staff member only is sufficient to supervise; other staff and students are to calmly resume their normal activities. When Kate comes out of her episode, she may need reminding of where she is. Kate is to return to her normal activities when she has settled, and she should remain at school.
- If required, Kate may take a 10-minute break in the sick bay or somewhere quiet. During this time, she is to use her strategies as listed above. After 10 minutes, Kate is to return to her normal activities.
- Kate should participate in normal school activities unless otherwise indicated.

Please do not hesitate to contact us for any queries.

Yours sincerely,

- — Signed by medical member of the team
- — Signed by allied health member of the team

Figure 13.2 School-based health care plan for Kate Jones.

In some situations the school-based health care plan needs to be overridden or changed. For students who experience *both* functional and epileptic seizures, the epileptic seizure plan always takes priority (and needs to be implemented) unless the school staff confidently recognise the occurrence of a *functional* seizure in any particular situation.

The school-based health care plan may also need to be *amended*, as in cases where the presentation of the functional seizures changes significantly over time. Such adjustments are typically straightforward because the school is continually monitoring the student and maintains ongoing contact with the health care team working with the young person (and family).

Graded Return to School (Partial Attendance)

Some young people, especially those who have been very unwell, may need a plan for a *graded return to school* (referred to, by educators, as *partial attendance*). Graded return to school can be helpful for students who have missed a significant amount of school, who have had a long history of untreated functional seizures, who have prolonged functional seizures, or who have multiple recurrent functional seizures in short time frames. The psychological and educational principles of a graded return to school are outlined below. Importantly, the time frame to achieve this goal varies greatly from one student to another. In general, it can usually be achieved within one or two school terms. The specifics of the graded return to school will need to be negotiated between the school, young person, family, and health care team using the principles outlined below. The plan should always take into account the young person's strengths and interests, so that the young person's motivation is kindled, facilitating a successful graded return to school.

- The initial goal is engagement in the school environment — including habituation of anxiety,[2] establishing feelings of safety, and establishing feelings of connection with others — rather than the completion of schoolwork. These baseline factors are necessary conditions for successful long-term learning and should be part of any plan for a graded return to school. Even if the student just sits in the classroom and begins to feel comfortable in the learning environment, this acclimation is an achievement in itself — the first step in the graded return to school. For some young people — especially those in primary school — acclimation and connection

---

2 *Habituation of anxiety* refers to the settling of anxiety over time — including physiological parameters of arousal — as the young person practises the anxiety-provoking activity time and time again.

with others can be facilitated by engagement in social activities (e.g., in small groups), handicraft activities, short meetings with supportive, 'safe' teachers, or doing some schoolwork they enjoy.

- Ideally, the plan for a graded return to school should include daily attendance for at least 1.5–2 hours, which should be enough for the student's anxiety about being at school to habituate. Attending school daily for these brief periods is better than attending full days once or twice a week. Daily attendance better approximates a student's normal timetable and offers more practice opportunities to manage anticipatory anxiety about returning to school. In many cases, the graded return can be accomplished over a relatively short time frame, in which the student would practise this first step for a two-week period and would then increase the time at school by another hour or two per day (as appropriate for that student). And so on, with the goal still being for the student to return to school full time — and not to get stuck in ongoing part-time attendance. For young people whose illness has been very severe or very long, the pace of the individualised return to school may need to be adjusted — lower and slower — to ensure a successful return to school.

- The majority of young people with functional seizures should be able to achieve full-time attendance. Necessary adjustments to the student's educational program — including adjustments relating to learning difficulties and psychological/social concerns such as the effects of anxiety on learning, difficulties managing academic pressure, and problems in maintaining healthy friendships — need to be addressed in a proactive, coordinated way. The time required to achieve full-time attendance varies greatly from one student to another. Usually (as noted above), one or two school terms is enough.

- In a small subset of young people — usually those whose functional seizures are complicated by significant and ongoing mental health concerns — only part-time attendance or an alternative, slower-stream schooling pathway may be feasible. In our own context in the state of New South Wales, Australia, the Higher School Certificate Pathways Program is one such example.

- The plan for a graded return to school should be regularly reviewed by the student, school, family, and health care team, with feedback from all members being used to revise and refine the plan as needed and to ensure that the student is progressing through the separate steps at an appropriate pace. Regular meetings between parents and the school can facilitate this process.

Development of an Individualised Learning Plan

Some young people may require the development of an ILP because they will struggle to manage the academic load on their return to school. The ILP addresses issues specific to that student and will again be negotiated through discussion with the student, school, family, and health care team. This ILP may require access to specialised support and additional funding (see below).

Special Considerations and Additional Funding

Many schools — and educational systems — have learning-support teams (or equivalent) that work to support students with additional needs, including those with illness or disability. In this context, schools frequently request a letter or report documenting that a young person has special needs or problems for the school to address — including, but not limited to, those addressed in the student's ILP. See Figure 13.3 for an example. This documentation is also potentially useful in efforts to secure additional supports to help address the student's special needs or problems. Our recommendation is that relevant documentation be included, when needed, as part of any plan for a graded return to school.

Problem-Solving with the School

Most schools will be able to implement, with no major difficulties, the clinical recommendations facilitating a return to school. Sometimes, however, schools need support in solving problems that arise. Below are some of the common problems or concerns that schools encounter, along with suggested ways of managing them:

The Opinion That the Young Person Should Not Return to School Before the Symptoms Are Gone

Sometimes the young person, a parent, or staff members at the school will voice the opinion — often in strong terms — that the young person should not or cannot return to school before the symptoms are gone and the young person has become well again. It is important to correct this misunderstanding and to explain that in the treatment of functional seizures — and functional neurological disorder, more broadly — attendance at school is part of the young person's treatment and that it facilitates the young person's recovery. In our team's

To Whom It May Concern:

Re Kate Jones

DOB 28.11.2009

Following our phone call today, I wanted to confirm that Kate Jones meets diagnostic criteria for the following:

1. Functional Neurological Symptom Disorder (Functional Seizure subtype)

2. Anxiety Disorder

These conditions have meant that Kate has missed a significant amount of schooling.

Part of the treatment for both of these conditions is a graded return to full-time school. We understand that the school has been very supportive in the past and would hope that the school could continue to support Kate. Some of the extra supports that Kate may require include: help with managing Kate's functional seizures should she have one at school (see school-based health plan for managing functional seizures), help with scaffolding her return to full-time schooling, and an individual learning support plan to help Kate catch up on school work she has missed out on.

Please do not hesitate to contact me should you have any further questions,

Yours sincerely

— Signed by Clinical Psychologist (or other member of the multidisciplinary team)

Figure 13.3 Funding letter for Kate Jones.

clinical experience, young people who do not return to school tend to have poorer outcomes, and their functional seizures are less likely to resolve than those who do return to school. In a nutshell, in medical terminology, not attending school is medically contraindicated.

Why the Young Person Should Return to School Instead of Doing Distance Learning

Sometimes either the school or the family will suggest distance education as an option for the young person. Our mind-body team strongly discourages distance learning, however, because attending the local school is both part of the treatment intervention for functional seizures and an outcome measure. Our team's clinical experience is that young people who do distance education or who do not go back to school do not have good outcomes. The negative effects of the loss of connection with the school — including the social relationships that are part of schooling — are also documented in the literature (Asadi-Pooya et al., 2021). Once again, the health care team may need to state explicitly, in writing, that distance learning is medically contraindicated for the young person.

The Concern That the Functional Seizures Will Be Distressing for Teachers and Other Students to Witness

Witnessing a functional seizure is typically distressing for anyone unfamiliar with them. At the outset, schools may need to organise a professional learning forum — what mental health clinicians call *psychoeducation* — about functional seizures for their staff. The central fact to be communicated is that functional seizures do not harm the young person. As a further step, and with parental consent, the school may want to consider meeting with the student's classmates or friends to raise awareness. For example, if a student is being supported by a group of friends, meeting with them to provide basic information about functional seizures — and to minimise secondary distress — is generally very helpful.

What to Do Regarding Young Persons Who Have Prolonged Functional Seizures

Although most functional seizures are relatively brief (less than 10 minutes in duration), some seizures last much longer than that — 20 to 60 minutes, possibly even longer. Different schools will have different capacities for managing these longer seizures, and these capacities may change over time as the school and its students adjust to witnessing the seizures. Another factor is that students experiencing the functional seizures will likely improve their capacities to avert the seizures altogether and to ride out the ones that do occur. In this context the school, family, and health care team should agree on a prearranged time limit specifying how long the school should be expected to manage a student's functional seizures. Having this sort of predefined time limit can help to ensure that the staff and students remain calm, knowing that the management of functional seizures that last longer than that will be escalated in one way or another. For example, the school might phone the parents to come and collect the student, or it might administer medication (as prescribed by the medical practitioner). As a background consideration, it should be remembered that the overarching aim is to keep the young persons at school and to avoid sending them home; as noted earlier, roughly 1.5–2 hours of daily school attendance is required for young persons' likely anxiety about being at school again to habituate.

The Young Person Does Not, or Is Unable to, Implement Regulation Strategies for Managing Functional Seizures

A very small number of young people struggle to manage their functional seizures (see Five-Step Plan in Chapter 6). These students may not be able to identify their warning signs or may not be able to use their regulation strategies to help manage their functional seizures. Even in such cases, however, the school can still use its established school-based health care plan to determine how it responds to the student's functional seizures.

The Parents Do Not Follow the School-Based Health Care Plan for Managing Functional Seizures

A very small number of parents struggle to follow the school-based plan for managing functional seizures. This is often due to their own anxiety regarding their child's functional seizures. These parents may struggle to send their child to school or may become distressed that their child is kept at school following a functional seizure. The first step in managing this problem is to have a joint meeting with the parents, school, and health care team to ensure that everyone is on the same page. Usually, these parental issues can be managed with further psychoeducation, additional coaching sessions with the parents (see Chapter 12), clarity about the school-based health care plan, and joint problem-solving around particular issues. Extremely rarely the parents will refuse to send the child to school, in which case the situation needs to be escalated to the department of education, with further dealings to be determined by the department's policies and processes regarding possible educational neglect.

What Happens If the Young Person Falls Hurting the Head?

While falls, and injuries secondary to falls, are not particularly common, they can be a feature of some presentations. To prevent falls and to keep the student safe, the school-based health care plans mandate that when students notice their warning signs of a functional seizure at school, they should — immediately — lower themselves down on the ground and implement their regulation strategies in an effort to down-regulate their arousal (calm down) and to avert the functional seizure.

If a fall does occur, then the school should follow its usual first-aid protocol around injuries at school.

Occasionally, when falls and potential injuries are recurrent parts of a student's presentation, our mind-body team has suggested temporary use of rugby helmets as a medical intervention to ensure that the student's head is protected. Given that falls are most likely when the student is moving from classroom to classroom, removing the helmet in class should be fine. And once the student has become more adept at reading the warning signs and at attaining a safe position — from which a fall is unlikely — the helmet will no longer be necessary.

Advocating for the Young Person and Family

In rare circumstances the family will encounter resistance from the school when negotiating the young person's return to school. Multiple reasons potentially underlie such resistance, including the following: a lack of understanding about functional seizures; a school-based health care plan that is insufficiently detailed to provide guidance for its implementation by the school; inadequate resources at the school to accommodate the student's emerging support needs; and a perception that the student's problems are too hard to manage.

In any of the above scenarios, it is part of the health care team's role to advocate for the family and young person at the school and to ensure that the young person's educational needs are met. The team needs to be clear that attendance at school is part of the young person's treatment plan and that staying at home or distance education would be detrimental to the young person's health and would delay or undermine the chances of recovery.

Importantly, principals and school staff may need time in advance to make appropriate plans and be prepared for the student's return. For this reason, it is important to ensure that school staff are provided with an estimated return-to-school date as soon as possible. In the meantime, if the original school remains resistant, the situation may need to be escalated to the appropriate department of education. In rare circumstances it may be necessary to locate an alternative school where the student's emerging support needs can be met.

Vignette: A Standard, Straightforward Integration into the Student's Local School

Raina was a 14-year-old girl who was referred to our Mind-Body Program for treatment of functional (stress) seizures. She had a history of epilepsy that had been well-managed with medications, and she had not had any epileptic seizures for the past four years. She had a long history of separation anxiety and generalised anxiety disorder. For example, even during sleepovers at her grand-parents' — with whom she was very close — she would become highly anxious. Raina would ruminate and worry constantly, particularly about schoolwork. She also had a learning disorder that had been unrecognised until the last year of primary school, meaning that she was far behind on her academic progress and in need of a high level of learning support. Raina had a six-month history of poor attendance at school, and because of the functional seizures, she had not attended school at all in the past two months. On school mornings, Raina would begin to tremble and shake. The trembling and shaking then progressed into multiple functional seizures, thereby frustrating her mother's attempts to drive Raina to school.

Raina completed the two-week Mind-Body Program. She learnt how to identify her warning signs for functional seizures and how to implement mind-body strategies to avert most of her functional seizures. Raina did extremely well in the structured hospital environment, including the hospital school. She also commenced taking medication for her severe, long-standing anxiety.

The mind-body team liaised closely with Raina's local school in order to prepare Raina and the school for her return to school. The following interventions were put in place within the school:

- We provided the local school with a school-based health care plan for managing Raina's functional seizures (which Raina had been practising in hospital).

- We problem-solved with the school on how to support Raina through some of her specific worries about returning to school. Raina was particularly worried about becoming lost at school and not being able to find her way to sickbay if needed. The school arranged for Raina to have a 'buddy' on her return to school. The buddy was there to support her socially, not to support her functional seizures, the latter being the responsibility of school staff. The school also arranged for the learning-support staff to meet Raina and her mother at the office on the first day of her return in order to help Raina transition to school.

- We suggested that the initial goal for Raina's return to school should be to practise being in the environment and letting her anxiety habituate rather than to engage with schoolwork. The school was happy to support this approach.

- Given Raina's high level of anxiety, we suggested a plan for her graded return to school, starting with half days before gradually increasing to full-time attendance over four weeks.

- We prescribed Raina PRN (*pro ray nata*, meaning 'as needed') medication to take on school mornings (short term) to help manage her anxiety (see Chapter 15 for medication options to help dampen high states of arousal).

- We coached Raina's mother on how to encourage and support Raina in returning to school despite the functional seizures. We also talked to the school about our expectations that Raina may initially have more-frequent functional seizures at school (triggered by her anxiety) but that we expected these to subside with habituation and also practice. The school was happy to support this effort to bring Raina to school — even knowing that some functional seizures would occur.

- The school had already put in place a learning-support program specifically to address Raina's learning difficulties.

With all of these supports in place, Raina and the school were able to manage her partial attendance at school. After the first week of attending, Raina's functional seizures had decreased to the point that she was no longer having any in the mornings before school. After five weeks of partial attendance, a small hiccup developed because Raina and her mother had settled into a routine of partial attendance. The school contacted our team at this point for support and recommendations about how to proceed. We met with Raina, her mother, and the school, and reframed the importance of Raina attending school full time as part of treating her anxiety and functional seizures. With this reframing, Raina was able to begin attending school full time.

Vignette: A Challenging and Difficult Integration Back into the Student's Local School

Evie was a 15-year-old girl who was in Year 10 at her local high school. She presented to the hospital with functional seizures that were triggered by pain. Evie's pain was called *precordial catch syndrome*. It involved sudden sharp pains that were very unpleasant — but not dangerous — and that occurred when Evie was stressed. When Evie experienced this pain and then, in turn, a functional seizure, she would collapse onto the ground and begin twitching and shaking, and still screaming in pain. During and after the functional seizure, Evie would experience high levels of emotional distress, and she vocalised her fears to all of those around her. Evie would yell, 'I am going to die!' or 'I can't take this anymore!' or 'Please just kill me!'

Understandably, when Evie experienced her pain and functional seizures in the school playground, the experience was very distressing for both students and staff. A number of Evie's peers became convinced that she was going to die and that the school was being punitive by following the school-based health care plan (which recommended minimal attention to the functional seizures). Some of Evie's peers were so distressed that they approached the school counsellor about this issue.

The school staff also had concerns about the emotional wellbeing of their staff and felt that in asking the staff to manage Evie's functional seizures at school, they were violating principles of occupational health and safety.

The school invited Evie's father to a meeting, where the staff outlined their concerns. The father became very distressed and raised his voice toward the school staff. The situation hit an impasse. Evie's father did not feel that it was fair for the school to exclude Evie from school because of her medical condition, and the school staff did not feel that they were equipped to manage Evie at school. In a parallel process, the more stressed the staff became and the more attention that was placed on Evie's functional seizures, the worse the seizures became (a negative cycle reinforcing the functional seizures). Attention to functional symptoms coupled with high arousal — the anxiety felt by the school staff — made them worse. The functional seizures began occurring more and more frequently at school and were lasting longer and longer.

Our mind-body team — which was trying to support the school — had to work hard to avoid becoming dragged into the tug-of-war between the school and Evie's father. In an effort to broaden the conversation, we asked for assistance from our hospital school staff, who had the advantage of being able to speak to Evie's school staff within an educational framework. In a joint meeting, we listened to the school's concerns and their anxieties about the emotional effect that Evie's functional seizures were having on staff and students. We supported the school in providing psychoeducation to their staff and students. We mediated a discussion between Evie, her father, and the school about what the school needed and what Evie needed.

The final agreement was as follows: the school placed some limits on Evie's activities on the school grounds. For example, she was not allowed in the playground at lunchtime until she could show that she could manage her functional seizures. Evie was also asked not to verbalise that she was going to die because this verbalisation made her friends (and other students) distressed. These interventions enabled the school staff to support Evie in managing her functional seizures, and the interventions also motivated Evie to use her strategies at school to manage her seizures. Slowly, the school and Evie began a positive cycle: as Evie was able to achieve better control over her functional seizures, the school was able to give her more freedom, which led to Evie having more positive experiences, and so on — establishing a positive cycle for increasing health and wellbeing.

Our mind-body team reviewed Evie's situation a year and a few months after we had finished our treatment intervention with her and her school. At that point, Evie had not had any functional seizures for 12 months. Moreover, she was delighted to report that the school had another student who suffered from functional seizures, which the school had managed with no difficulties. In fact, there were now posters around the school advising staff on how to respond to functional seizures.

Step 1: Engagement with the school

Engagement with the school as part of the biopsychosocial assessment. The school becomes a member of the multidisciplinary team.

Step 2: Development of a school-based health care plan for managing functional seizures, along with personalised learning support

The health care team, family, student, and school staff collaborate to develop a school-based health care plan, along with any adjustments that the student may need in personalised learning support.

Step 3: Problem solving

The health care team, family, student, and school staff problem-solve any issues that could potentially disrupt or complicate the young person's return to school.

Step 4: Updating the school-based health care plan and personalised learning support

The health care team, the family, the student, and school staff collaborate to review, when needed, the school-based health care plan and learning-support plan (with the consequence that these plans do not remain static but can continue to evolve as the student recovers).

Figure 13.4 Health care team collaboration with the school. This flowchart provides a visual representation of the health care team's engagement with the school.
© Kasia Kozlowska and Blanche Savage 2022

Summing Up

To bring this long chapter into focus, we provide a flowchart of the health care team's engagement with the school (Figure 13.4) and a summary of the key challenges for schools in learning to manage students' functional seizures (Text Box 13.1).

Text Box 13.1
In a Nutshell: Learning to Manage Functional Seizures in the School Setting

A close and collaborative relationship with the school is key to a successful outcome—the young person with functional seizures returning to normal function and full-time schooling.

To manage a functional seizure, each school will need to be clear about the following elements:

- What will happen if a student has a functional seizure at school (from the school-based health care plan for managing functional seizures)?
- Who will supervise the student?
- What will happen to the other students in the class?
- What factors might require an escalation or emergency response (e.g., administration of medication if the functional seizure continues for >60 minutes)?
- At what point will the student's parents be called?

The school-based health care plan will continually evolve with input from the health care team, family, student, and school staff to meet the student's changing needs as the student improves in health and wellbeing and as the functional seizures decrease or even no longer occur.

Chapter 14

Working with the Medical Team: The Young Person with Comorbid Medical or Functional Conditions

In this chapter, we briefly review some of the comorbid medical and functional conditions that may require treatment from the family doctor, the general paediatrician, a paediatric neurologist or other specialist. The most common medical and functional conditions that are encountered in young people with functional seizures include the following: epileptic seizures; postural orthostatic intolerance and postural orthostatic tachycardia syndrome (POTS) (van der Zalm et al., 2019; Wells et al., 2018); and functional gut disorders (Hyams et al., 2016). Because all these conditions may complicate the clinical picture and require treatment by a medical professional — alongside the treatment of functional seizures (or other comorbid functional neurological symptoms) — we discuss each briefly in the sections below.

Working with Young People Who Suffer from Epilepsy and Functional Seizures

Some young people have both epileptic and functional seizures. As a mental health clinician, you will need to work closely with the young person's neurologist (or epilepsy team), who should provide a school-based health care plan for managing the young person's epileptic seizures (separate from any plan for her[1] functional seizures). Although this handbook is appropriate for working with and managing the young person's functional seizures, it cannot be used to manage the epileptic seizures, which require a different treatment. In this context, the young person's school-based health care plan for functional seizures should be explicit in how to differentiate between epileptic and functional seizures.

---

1 As noted in earlier chapters, because functional somatic symptoms occur more frequently in girls than in boys, we generally use the pronouns she and her to reflect this clinical reality.

On the one hand, when family members, teachers, or other adults (i.e., whoever might be present when a seizure occurs) are able to distinguish between the young person's epileptic and functional seizures, the school-based health care plan is straightforward. An epileptic seizure activates the school-based health care plan for epileptic seizures, and a functional seizure activates the school-based health care plan for functional seizures (see Chapter 13). A 24-hour video electroencephalogram (vEEG) can assist both professionals and families in learning to distinguish the two types of seizure events (Tatum et al., 2022; Whitehead et al., 2017).

On the other hand, if family members, teachers, or other adults have not yet learned to distinguish between the young person's epileptic and functional seizures, the school-based health care plan for epileptic seizures must always take precedence. In the meantime — that is, until those present are able to distinguish between seizure types — the clinician and young person can continue to work on identifying the warning signs for functional seizures and practising regulation strategies at regular intervals during the day.

Below we provide an example of a combined school-based health care plan for a student with both epileptic and functional seizures in the school setting (see Figure 14.1).

Postural Orthostatic Intolerance and Postural Orthostatic Tachycardia Syndrome

An important finding from the research associated with our Mind-Body Program was that young people with functional seizures show activation and dysregulation of their autonomic nervous system (Chudleigh et al., 2019; Kozlowska, Palmer, et al., 2015). In this context it is not surprising that many of them have comorbid mental health or functional somatic symptoms that reflect activation and dysregulation of the autonomic system.[2] Postural orthostatic intolerance and POTS, which present as dizziness or fainting on standing, involve too little restorative parasympathetic activity (allowing heart rate to increase) and too much sympathetic activity (through which heart rate increases even more on standing). Blood pressure remains stable.

A diagnosis of POTS should be made by a medical practitioner because there are multiple reasons why a young person may experience dizziness and fainting. A standing test on waking — where the young person's heart rate and blood pressure are monitored each minute for ten minutes — is a useful test. In young

---

2 For a detailed discussion of the autonomic system, see Chapter 6 of Kozlowska, Scher, and Helgeland (2020). For a summary of research studies and biomarker changes, see Online Supplement 6.1 (part of the same book).

Jane Doe Health Care Plan for Managing Seizures in the School Setting:

Clinical Presentation with Both Epileptic and Functional Seizures

Seizure Management Plan for Jane Doe

Jane Doe presents with both epileptic and functional seizures. Jane is on anti-seizure medications. This is a health-care plan for her epileptic seizures and for her functional seizures.

Epileptic Seizures

Jane's epileptic seizures are stereotyped and involve walking in circles before dropping to the floor and having generalised tonic-clonic jerking.

In the event that Jane has a generalised tonic-clonic seizure (loss of awareness, body stiffening, eyes open and deviated, with lips going blue ± jerking of one or more limbs), you should:

1. Stay calm.

2. Time the event.

3. Stay with Jane and position her on her side in the recovery position.

4. Provide comfort, reassurance, and a safe environment.

5. Check for breathing.

6. Don't put anything in her mouth.

7. When the epileptic seizures stops, allow Jane to sleep or rest.

If the epileptic seizure is still going at five minutes, call for an ambulance (by dialling the local emergency number [000 in Australia]), AND give 10 mg (2 vial of 5 mg/ml) of midazolam buccal/intranasal as instructed.

If the epileptic seizure has stopped by the time the ambulance has arrived, and if Jane has recovered and her mother or other relative is present, she can go home with them rather than being taken to hospital to recover further.

Functional Seizures

Jane's functional seizures involve her staring blankly into the distance and being unresponsive to people around her

Jane's early warning signs for a functional seizure are the following:

1. Feeling a pounding heart

2. Feeling butterflies in her stomach

3. Feeling dizzy

If Jane notices her early warning signs, she should get on the floor and practise her regulation strategies, which include the following:

- Slow breathing

- Using her fidget toys

- Listening to music

If Jane has a functional seizure:

- An ambulance does not need to be called. Functional seizures are not dangerous.

continued over page ...

- Ensure that she is safe and that she will not hit her head.

- Only one person needs to monitor her.

Following a functional seizure:

- Jane may need to be reminded where she is.
- She can use her regulation strategies to help her calm down (5–10 minutes).
- Jane should then return to the activities she was doing before her functional seizure.

If you are unsure whether Jane is having an epileptic or a functional seizure, the health care plan for epileptic seizures must take precedence.

Yours sincerely

Dr Smith
Neurologist

Figure 14.1 Example of a school-based health care plan for managing both epileptic and functional seizures.

people, a stable blood pressure coupled with an increase in heart rate of >40 beats per minute is consistent with POTS. An increase in heart rate that does not reach over 40 beats per minute but that is accompanied by significant symptoms is considered postural orthostatic intolerance. Treatment of these forms of orthostatic intolerance is important because the symptoms complicate many presentations of functional seizures.

Treatment for POTS includes the following elements:

- Good hydration throughout the day

- Sufficient consumption of salt with meals (or salt supplements)

- Use of supportive leggings

- Getting up out of bed incrementally: sitting up first, waiting for the body (autonomic system) to settle, then standing

- Use of mind-body strategies that help regulate the autonomic nervous system (e.g., slow breathing in the sitting state before getting out of bed)

- Regular exercise to help regulate the autonomic nervous system (POTS commonly develops in the context of bedrest [e.g., following an illness])

- In POTS that is severe and does not respond to the above measures, medications can be trialled (see Chapter 15 for further information pertaining to medications)

Because postural orthostatic intolerance and postural orthostatic tachycardia syndrome caused by activation and dysregulation of the autonomic system (absence of an organic cause) are functional disorders, many paediatricians are not familiar with their management. Provision of educational resources can be helpful (Kozlowska, Scher, & Helgeland, 2020; Rowe, 2014; van der Zalm et al., 2019; Wells et al., 2018).

Functional Gut Symptoms

The gut is regulated by the brain-gut-microbiota axis. The autonomic system is part of this axis. Consequently, functional gut disorders, such as functional constipation, functional abdominal pain, symptoms of irritable bowel, functional nausea, and so on, are common comorbid symptoms in young people with functional seizures. When certain symptoms become problematic — for example, functional constipation — careful management by a family doctor or paediatrician is helpful. For further information, including the use of medication to treat functional gut symptoms, see Chapter 10 of Kozlowska, Scher, and Helgeland (2020).

Chapter 15

Medication as an Adjunct to Treatment

According to the Stress-System Model for functional somatic symptoms that we use to frame our work, functional seizures involve excessive activation of brain stress systems — in response to physical, emotional, relational, or academic stress — and dysregulation of neural (brain) networks. The treatment of functional seizures involves the use of mind-body regulation strategies that help young persons to down-regulate (switch off) the stress system and increase their capacity to manage the challenges of daily living. The treatment may also include psychosocial interventions that address stress in the environment. In this chapter, we discuss a range of medications that are sometimes used as an adjunct — most typically, as a *temporary* adjunct — during the treatment intervention. Importantly, there is no medication for functional seizures per se. When used, medications target specific factors that contribute to the young person's presentation: sleep disturbance, high arousal levels, overwhelming anxiety, or comorbid mental health concerns. They need to be carefully monitored and then discontinued if they have no useful effect or when they are no longer needed. Medications are never used alone. They are always used alongside other therapeutic interventions (see Chapters 6, 7, 9, 10, 12).

Medications are prescribed by a medical practitioner — the family doctor, paediatrician, or child and adolescent psychiatrist who is part of the multidisciplinary treating team. In the following sections we briefly mention the adjunct medications that we most frequently use in our Mind-Body Program. The material about melatonin, clonidine, and quetiapine is adapted, with slight modifications, from Online Supplement 5.1 of Kozlowska, Scher, and Helgeland, Functional Somatic Symptoms in Children and Adolescents: A Stress-System Approach to Assessment and Treatment (2020), published under the terms of the Creative Commons Attribution-NonCommercial-NoDerivatives 4.0 International License (http://creativecommons.org /licenses/by-nc-nd/4.0/).

We also note that because we expect that psychiatrists and other medical doctors will be the ones determining whether to use medications as an adjunct to other treatments, the detailed information we provide here is geared primarily toward that particular subset of health care professionals. Other health care professionals should look to obtain an overview of medication use and an understanding of the range of factors that go into determining medication use for this particular patient population.

Medications for Sleep

Disrupted sleep is a common symptom of stress-system activation. Sleep disruption appears to be caused by increased activity of the sympathetic system (causing arousals from sleep) and dysregulation in cortisol secretion (also disrupting the sleep/wake cycle) (Chung et al., 2022).[1] Because regulation of sleep has such a substantial impact on the young person's health and wellbeing and on the capacity to heal, our mind-body team gives particular attention to regulating the circadian clock — which is typically our first intervention, implemented at the very beginning of the treatment program.

The sleep intervention always includes behavioural interventions: scheduling sleep at the right time, exposure to sun or bright light in the morning, good sleep hygiene, shutting down computer screens well before bedtime, and so on (Kozlowska, Scher, & Helgeland, 2020). For young people whose sleep is very disturbed, our mind-body team sometimes uses adjunct medication — on a temporary basis — to help regulate the circadian clock. Below we discuss our most commonly used interventions.[2]

Melatonin

Melatonin, a hormone produced by the pineal gland at bedtime, regulates sleep and wakefulness (Schwartz & Goradia, 2013). If sleep initiation is the problem, melatonin 3–9 mg immediate-release preparation can be trialled. The 3 mg dose is always trialled first. If sleep maintenance is the problem, melatonin 2–8 mg slow-release preparation can be trialled. The 2 mg dose is always trialled first. Melatonin immediate-release and slow-release preparations can be used in combination if needed. Melatonin can also be combined with any of the medications below.

---

1 For more information see Chapter 5 about the circadian clock in Kozlowska, Scher, and Helgeland (2020).

2 For other options not discussed in this chapter, see Online Supplement 5.1 of Kozlowska, Scher, and Helgeland (2020).

Clonidine

Clonidine helps to down-regulate (switch off) the brain stress systems, and it can be helpful in managing trauma-related nightmares. A nonselective alpha-2 agonist, the medication has an overall inhibitory action primarily at adrenergic alpha-2 autoreceptors (it stimulates the brake) of the locus coeruleus. The locus coeruleus gives rise to a mass of noradrenaline-containing projections throughout the brain, including the amygdala. Through its alpha-2 agonist activity, clonidine reduces catecholamine (stress hormone) levels (Wilson et al., 2017; Stahl, 2021) (see Figure 15.1). Its action on imidazoline receptors is thought to be responsible for some of its sedating effects (Ernsberger & Haxhiu, 1997). Clonidine 0.025 mg (i.e., one-fourth of 0.1 mg tablet titrated up to 0.1 mg depending on response and weight) at bedtime can be especially helpful if the young person has a very high level of arousal at night (including trauma-related nightmares or flashbacks). Clonidine can be combined with melatonin. Because clonidine lowers blood pressure, a small number of young people may be unable to tolerate it or may be able to tolerate only a small dose. For this reason, the starting dose is always very small and titrated up by small increments of 0.025 mg. If tolerated, the longer-term side effects are minimal. Clonidine tablets are soluble in water if doses smaller than 0.025 mg are required (Burridge & Symons, 2018).

Quetiapine

Quetiapine is an atypical antipsychotic approved by the US Food and Drug Administration for treating bipolar disorder, schizophrenia, and generalised anxiety disorder, and as an adjunct treatment for treatment-resistant depression. Quetiapine is sedating, dampens cortical arousal, and promotes sleep and normalisation of sleep architecture via a complex combination of mechanisms (Schwartz & Goradia, 2013). An accumulating evidence base supports the use of quetiapine as a neuromodulator in chronic pain conditions and as a useful medication for stabilising sleep in patients with chronic pain or with other functional somatic symptoms (Tornblom & Drossman, 2018) (see Tornblom and Drossman [2018] for a review of studies). Most patients with functional somatic symptoms can be helped with very small doses of quetiapine (6.25–37.5 mg total, per day). Unpleasant dreams or nightmares are rare side effects. Because of quetiapine's potential for weight gain and metabolic side effects, we use it as an interim measure only (usually up to three months). Once sleep has stabilised and the young person's function has improved, the quetiapine can be gradually withdrawn, generally free of complications. Quetiapine can be combined with melatonin or clonidine. The use of quetiapine is off-label and is typically reserved for young people who are very ill — and only in low doses as an interim measure.

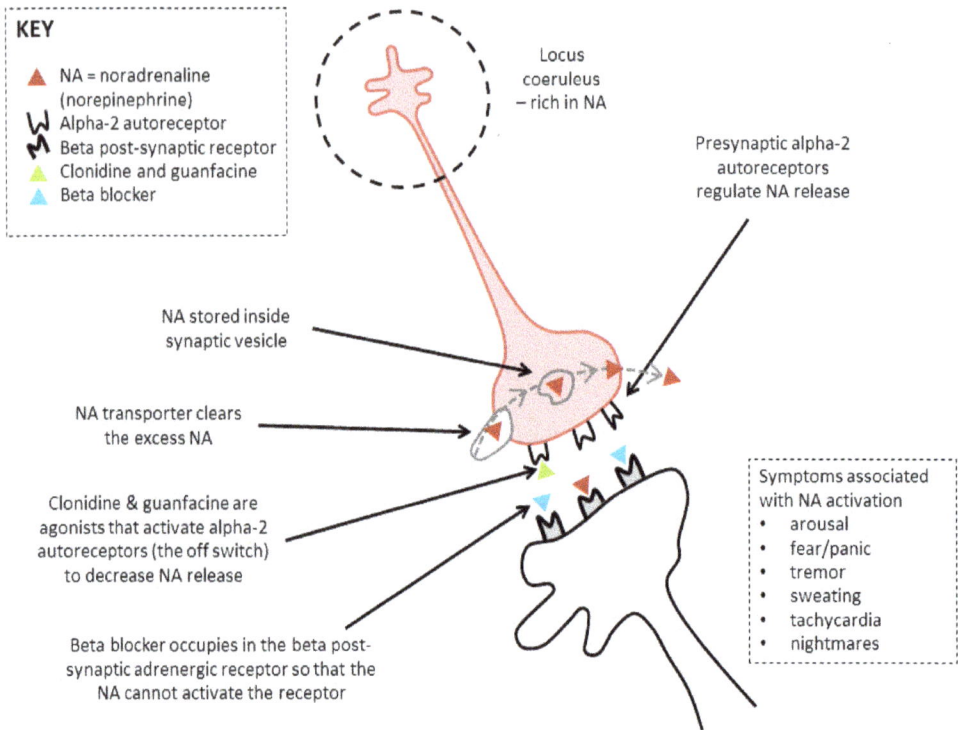

KEY

▲ NA = noradrenaline (norepinephrine)
Ⱳ Alpha-2 autoreceptor
Ⱳ Beta post-synaptic receptor
▲ Clonidine and guanfacine
▲ Beta blocker

Locus coeruleus – rich in NA

Presynaptic alpha-2 autoreceptors regulate NA release

NA stored inside synaptic vesicle

NA transporter clears the excess NA

Clonidine & guanfacine are agonists that activate alpha-2 autoreceptors (the off switch) to decrease NA release

Beta blocker occupies in the beta post-synaptic adrenergic receptor so that the NA cannot activate the receptor

Symptoms associated with NA activation
• arousal
• fear/panic
• tremor
• sweating
• tachycardia
• nightmares

Figure 15.1 Therapeutic actions of clonidine, guanfacine, and beta blockers. Noradrenergic neurons mediating brain arousal from the locus coeruleus. The locus coeruleus is the main source of noradrenaline synthesis in the brain. It reaches upward, forward, and downward, sending projections throughout the brain. Clonidine and guanfacine are agonists that activate alpha-2 autoreceptors (the off switch) to decrease noradrenalin release. Beta blockers occupy the beta post-synaptic adrenergic receptor, effectively blocking it so that the noradrenalin cannot activate the receptor.
© Kasia Kozlowska 2022

Medications That Help Modulate Arousal

A subset of young people with functional seizures are initially in a state of such high arousal that they struggle to learn, practise, and implement any of the regulation strategies that we discuss in this manual. Young people from this group may be experiencing numerous functional seizures throughout the day, or their functional seizures may be prolonged (lasting for hours at a time). In this difficult-to-treat scenario, our mind-body team may trial some medications — on a temporary basis (usually 3–6 months) — that help decrease the young person's arousal, thereby creating space for the young person to engage with the treatment program. The long-term goal is for the young person to manage neurophysiological regulation using regulation strategies without pharmacotherapy. If medication is to be used, we would suggest trialling medication sooner rather than later, thereby providing the young person with the best chance of breaking the cycle of functional somatic symptoms (including functional seizures).

Propranolol

Propranolol, commonly known as a *beta blocker*, is a beta-adrenoceptor antagonist that blocks beta-adrenergic receptors in body tissues and in the central nervous system (see Figure 15.1). Adrenergic receptors are the targets of catecholamines — adrenaline (epinephrine) and noradrenaline (norepinephrine) — which are released in response to stress-related sympathetic activation of the adrenal glands. These two catecholamines function as *stress hormones in the body* and as *arousal-promoting (stress system) neurotransmitters in the brain*. In young people with functional seizures, propranolol can be used to target a number of different arousal-related processes.

On the body-system level, propranolol can be used to target beta-adrenergic receptors located in the heart, blood vessels, and sweat glands, all of which are activated when the sympathetic component of the autonomic nervous system is switched on, leading to the release of adrenaline and noradrenalin from the adrenal glands. Propranolol blocks these beta-adrenergic receptors to attenuate episodes of extreme sympathetic activation that occur in the context of panic attacks or orthostatic intolerance/postural orthostatic tachycardia syndrome (POTS) (see Chapter 14).

On the brain-system level, propranolol can be used to block beta-adrenergic receptors activated by noradrenaline, the brain's key catecholamine — arousal-mediating neurotransmitter — that activates in the context of stress and the challenges of daily living (Arnsten, 2015; Wilson et al., 2017). Because propranolol is lipophilic — that is, it dissolves in fat — it can cross the blood-brain barrier and act on beta-adrenergic receptors in the brain (Wilson et al., 2017). And because children and adolescents with functional seizures (vs. healthy controls) show a greater degree of cortical arousal in response to stress (Braun et al., 2021; Radmanesh et al., 2020), propranolol can be used to help attenuate the young person's arousal, thereby providing the young person with a therapeutic window in which to practise her regulation strategies (see, e.g., the case of BJ (Ratnamohan et al., 2018)).

Alongside the above-described effects, propranolol may disrupt both the formation of fear conditioning and the reconsolidation of fear memories (Stahl, 2021).

Propanolol is given on a morning and afternoon dosage schedule (beginning at a dose of 2.5 mg and potentially titrated up to 5 mg, 7.5 mg, or 10 mg). It is not taken at night because it can disrupt the circadian clock.

Propranolol is contraindicated in young people with asthma because the ongoing activation of beta-2 adrenergic receptors in the smooth muscle of the lungs maintains vasodilation; blockage of these receptors by propranolol may constrict smooth muscle and worsen asthma symptoms.

Clonidine

As noted above, clonidine helps to down-regulate (switch off) the brain stress systems, decreasing arousal (see Figure 15.1). Clonidine can be used in very small doses throughout the day to help dampen young persons' arousal while they learn their self-regulation strategies. Plasma levels of clonidine peak within 30–60 minutes of oral administration, with a half-life of 5–13 hours (and potentially even longer) — meaning that it provides some assistance over that period of time.

Guanfacine

Guanfacine is a selective alpha-2A adrenergic agonist that, like clonidine, helps to down-regulate (switch off) the brain stress systems and decrease arousal (see Figure 15.1). In addition, emerging research suggests that guanfacine may influence dendritic spine plasticity and neuronal network connectivity in the prefrontal cortex (Huss et al., 2016), potentially facilitating the improved self-regulation hoped to be achieved through treatment. Guanfacine MR (modified release) is the only dosage form available in Australia. Guanfacine MR has a long half-life and is taken once a day. The starting dose is 1 mg. For young people with functional seizures — or other difficult-to-treat functional neuro-logical symptoms (e.g., fixed dystonia) — our mind-body team has used doses of 1 mg to 7 mg. We typically prescribe it at night, but some children prefer to take it in the morning.

Prazosin

High levels of noradrenalin are released during acute stress or when a young person is experiencing posttraumatic symptoms (hyperarousal, insomnia, and trauma-related nightmares) (Arnsten et al., 2015). Prazosin, a lipid-soluble alpha-1 adrenoceptor blocker, blocks post-synaptic alpha-1 receptors that bind noradrenalin and are activated by it. When treating young persons with trauma-related nightmares, prazosin can be given in bedtime doses of 1–4 mg (Akinsanya et al., 2017). A small daytime dose can also reduce arousal symptoms during the day. Our mind-body team has trialled prazosin when more commonly used medications (e.g., propranolol, clonidine, and guanfacine) have failed to settle young persons with functional seizures and posttraumatic stress disorder. For this particular group of patients, hyperarousal is so very marked that it undermines both the restorative functions of sleep and the young persons' efforts to implement regulation strategies. Combinations of prazosin and propranolol are usually avoided or are monitored very carefully for possible drops in blood pressure.

Medications for Comorbid Nausea or Constipation

Because young people with functional neurological disorder (including functional seizures) show activation or dysregulation of the autonomic nervous system (Chudleigh et al., 2019; Kozlowska, Palmer, et al., 2015), they often suffer from comorbid functional gut symptoms that reflect this activation/dysregulation.[3] Nausea reflects activation of the defensive arm of the parasympathetic system. Constipation reflects activation of the sympathetic system, which shuts down gut function. And orthostatic intolerance/POTS (discussed above and in Chapter 14) reflects too little restorative parasympathetic (vagal) activity (allowing heart rate to increase) and too much sympathetic activity (through which the heart rate increases even more), with no change in blood pressure. Orthostatic intolerance/POTS is sometimes accompanied by nausea on standing, reflecting concurrent activation of the defensive arm of the parasympathetic system.

When gut-related symptoms are extreme — and they affect the young person's capacity to engage in the treatment — they may need to be treated in their own right.

Nausea

Nausea is a common symptom experienced by young people with functional neurological disorder (including functional seizures). Ondansetron can be used as an anti-nausea medication. Ondansetron is available as a tablet, liquid, or wafers (which dissolve when placed under the tongue). Ondansetron is a highly selective serotonin receptor (SHT3) antagonist. The exact mechanism of action in the treatment of nausea (and vomiting) is unclear, but it is known to block the effect of serotonin on the vomiting centre in the medulla.

Constipation

Constipation, also a common comorbidity for functional neurological disorder (including functional seizures), can be treated with various medications.

---

3 For a detailed discussion of neurobiology, see Chapter 6 of Kozlowska, Scher, and Helgeland (2020).

Options include osmotic laxatives (e.g., lactulose), iso-osmotic laxatives (e.g., macrogol [Movicol, Osmolax)], stool softeners (dioctyl sodium sulfosuccinate [Coloxyl] and senna), and various fibre preparations. Adolescents sometimes forget to drink enough, causing mild dehydration, constipation, and headaches.

Medications for Comorbid Anxiety and Depression

As discussed in Chapter 11, the rate of comorbid mental health conditions in young people with functional neurological disorder (including functional seizures) — most commonly, depression or anxiety — varies widely (22%–80% of children and adolescents in different cohorts) (Vassilopoulos et al., 2022). In the experience of our mind-body team, the resolution of both functional seizures and comorbid mental health concerns substantially improves long-term health and wellbeing (Kozlowska, Gray, et al., 2020). In this context, some young people with functional seizures and comorbid mental health conditions may also require treatment with a combination of psychotherapy and medication. The selective serotonin reuptake inhibitors (SSRIs) are the class of medications that we most often use for anxiety and depression (Hetrick et al., 2021). Our key recommendations in treating young people with functional seizures — and functional disorders more generally — are to (1) start with very small doses and to increase very slowly to the lowest therapeutic dose,[4] in order to avoid side effects, (2) communicate to the young person that the medication will begin to work approximately six weeks after the therapeutic dose is reached (i.e., that the medication does not work immediately); and (3) highlight that medication works best when coupled with psychotherapy to reduce relapse and to increase compliance.

---

4 For example, when using fluoxetine, we commonly start with a dose of 2.5 mg in the morning and increase every 5-10 days by 2.5 mg until reaching the therapeutic dose of 20 mg in the morning. This approach takes into account that fluoxetine and its breakdown products have a very long half-life.

Chapter 16

A Young Person's Lived Experience, and Some Further Reflections

We open this concluding chapter with a reflection from Bernadette, a 14-year-old adolescent girl. When Bernadette heard that we were writing a clinician manual for functional seizures, she offered to share her personal experience of the therapeutic process and her own journey of working with us (BS and KK) and the mind-body team more generally. Her reflection touches upon the role of hope and positive expectations (discussed in Chapter 9), the importance of listening to the body and understanding its somatic narrative (discussed in Chapter 7), the need to shift focus-of-attention from the symptoms to the implementation of mind-body strategies (discussed in Chapters 6, 9, and 10), and the necessity of reflecting about one's own story and understanding the factors that have come together to activate the body and to drive the illness process (Chapter 3). The reflection also highlights the need to be creative. With the support of the mind-body team, Bernadette was able to devise her own plan for managing functional seizures. She used a *four Rs* acronym to do this: recognise, release, reframe, and regulate. In our clinical practice, the mind-body team always supports young persons' efforts to devise interventions for functional seizures that work for them. In doing so we are strengthening their sense of mastery and control — key elements of the pathway to health.

Bernadette's Reflection: The Lived Experience of Functional Seizures and the Therapeutic Process

In Bernadette's own words:

> Overcoming functional seizures is hard and can cause a lot of doubt. Doubts about not knowing when things will reach some form of 'normality' and, I imagine in some cases, if the seizures will ever go away. In these times, it is really important to have faith — the

banishment of doubt — because it gives you something to hold onto during this challenging time. But faith can only bring you so far.

I think it is important to get to the root cause of these symptoms so that you don't just cover it with a bandaid and not address the actual problem. This isn't putting a label on what you have. It is about addressing your unique and individual problem and finding out what that is. I say 'problem' for the lack of a better word.

For example, the root cause of my symptoms was my tendency to put pressure on myself. I just challenged myself so much that I eventually burnt out. By acknowledging and accepting what caused the symptoms, I was able to make changes in my everyday life to stop my functional seizures and stop them from evolving and changing into another symptom.

The first step to helping with functional seizures is to acknowledge that the mind and body aren't separate and are in fact one entity. This influences the idea that you need to listen to the body and not override the signals it provides. The language of the mind is through words, and the language of the body is through sensations, emotions, and feelings.

Also, finding the right balance comes into play a lot, like when finding the right balance between focusing on symptoms versus focusing on strategies. Think about it this way. Once you recognise what your body is trying to communicate to you, release and let go of the sensations/feelings that have come up. Then reframe those sensations/feelings and look at them from a different perspective. Remember, there is no good or bad sensation/feeling. And then put your regulation strategies in place. I remembered what to do using the four Rs: recognise, release, reframe, and regulate.

For me, I found it really difficult to recognise the signals my body gave me before transitioning into a functional seizure. But, even when I finally started to recognise and identify how I felt, I would override my feelings and carry on. Here, you also need to find the right balance between listening to your mind and your body. It is good to use rational and common sense, but your body's instincts and feelings have a really important role, too. So, listen to your body.

When I was about to slip into a functional seizure, my ears would begin to ring and block up. For other people it might be that their throat tightens, their stomach squelches, or they develop a headache.

With this, it is different for everybody, and no 'one size fits all', so you need to understand your body and recognise what works for you.

The next steps didn't come so hard to me, but they are still very important. In the next step, you really need to take into consideration the balance between recognising your symptoms and implementing your strategies. Once you notice that your symptoms are flaring up, you can put in place your strategies to stop the functional seizure, which again can be very different for everyone. It took me months of practice to master this step.

In summary, overcoming functional seizures is hard, but you can definitely return to life without them. It comes down to having faith, identifying why you are seizing, changing your lifestyle, and having a clear functional seizure plan that you put into action when you can feel yourself slipping into a functional seizure. And as I mentioned before, what worked for me may not work for you, so don't be disheartened if this doesn't work. Just remember to persevere and have faith.

Concluding Reflections from the Authors

Some three years ago, we — the first and last author — decided to summarise in writing all that we had learnt from our research and from our work with patients (and their families) about treating children and adolescents with functional seizures. We had come a long way. Nearly three decades ago, the team as it was then — the last author (KK) is the only remaining member — cared for an adult-sized adolescent boy with frequent, violent functional seizures. To protect him from falling from his bed onto the floor, we moved his mattress onto the floor. And not having any reliable idea about how to treat his functional seizures, we did the best we could: we enrolled him in our Mind-Body Program and used the program's therapeutic elements to try to settle him down and restore normal function. After a longish and difficult admission, he was able to return home and go back to his local school. Many years later his mother contacted the team to let us know that he had been accepted into medical school. In our conversation she was surprised (and delighted) that KK remembered all the details of her son's story: all the stressors (adverse childhood experiences) that had triggered his presentation.

Since that time, through clinical observation, numerous research projects, creative problem-solving, and well-informed hunches, our mind-body team has developed what we consider a good enough treatment program. We say good enough because we hold Donald Winnicott's idea of the 'good enough parent' close to heart. Through the trials and tribulations of working with different patients and their families — sometimes trying to manage symptoms that refused to settle — we have always held this idea in mind and close to our hearts. The *good-enough* position means trusting the innate healing capacities of the human body. We took the position that the body's healing capacities, coupled with the power of the therapeutic relationship, the clinical skills of our mind-body team, and the team's determination to identify workable solutions to whatever problems arose, would generate good outcomes. And as these efforts continued over time, we were confident that we could develop and consolidate a treatment program that would help most young people most of the time.

Over the last decade, our team has become increasingly aware of the need for clinical resources for mental health clinicians to use in the treatment of young people with functional seizures. We receive an ongoing trickle of emails and phone calls from clinicians around Australia asking for help and clinical support. At times the trickle becomes a flood. Repeatedly, mental health clinicians have told us that training to address functional seizures — and functional somatic symptoms more generally — was never part of their university and postgraduate education. As a consequence, the prospect of treating functional seizures has typically been experienced as unsettling, anxiety provoking, overwhelming, or even scary. And it has certainly been perceived as being outside of the mental health clinician's scope of practice. Cumulatively, these ongoing requests put increasing pressure on us to share what we had learnt, and they also, in turn, sparked the idea of writing this manual.

Stories told by families — portraying their convoluted paths through the medical system as they sought to obtain help — highlighted that health care systems remain seriously deficient in identifying, assessing, and treating young people with functional neurological disorder (FND), including functional seizures (Kozlowska et al., 2021). The stories highlighted the need to educate clinicians, disseminate and integrate research findings into clinical practice, and change an outdated culture of care (Kozlowska et al., 2021). Our own experience of young people with FND and their families is that they are open to working with clinicians in a collaborative way and that they are generous in their contributions to research. They want to know and understand what is going on. Many children and adolescents have unsparingly contributed to our research program, which, in turn — based on a growing body of research findings — has enabled us to develop and integrate more effective, targeted interventions into our treatment program. Of course, this process of translating research findings into clinical practice is ongoing.

During the current COVID-19 pandemic, the need for clinical resources on FND, including functional seizures, has become even more apparent. Our team and the paediatricians we work with have noted a sharp increase in children and adolescents presenting with these problems. For example, in Australia and around the world, the number of distressed adolescent girls presenting with late-onset functional tics has jumped dramatically (Han et al., 2022; Heyman et al., 2021; Pringsheim et al., 2021). And in the young people that we worked with, we observed that the tics often morphed into, or co-existed with, functional seizures (a shift in symptoms being a common feature of paediatric FND). Our Mind-Body Program has been overwhelmed by the numbers, and we were unable to respond to the need for prompt assessment and treatment. Our waitlist for an assessment — usually carried out in a timely way — is much longer than ever before.

By hook or by crook, we have, during this stressful time of COVID-19, eked out the time required to produce this manual. We also reached out to colleagues from around the world — some of whom we had met before and some of whom we connected with through their publications or through other colleagues — to help us disseminate this manual by translating (pro bono) the Fact Sheet (Appendix B) and Five-Step Plan (see Appendixes C and D) into their native languages. When the reader accesses the manual's website at Australian Academic Press, they will find these resources available in an ever-growing number of languages; we plan on adding more as new translations become available. This willingness of our colleagues to contribute to the manual, to make it more user-friendly for clinicians and their patients in non–English speaking countries — during a time when they were also overwhelmed with the stress of the COVID-19 pandemic — has not only been affirming but has highlighted the growing momentum behind by mental health clinicians' determination to work together to change the culture of care.

As the reader knows, in this manual we have tried to outline the steps that mental health clinicians need to take to treat young people with functional seizures. Because it is difficult to keep the entire process in mind, we thought it useful to provide you, the clinician, with a flowchart (Figure 16.1) that summarises the therapeutic processes summarised in this manual. The flowchart is designed to function as a road map that you can consult when you feel lost or when the next step in the therapeutic process is difficult to see. A printout version of the flowchart is available as Appendix G.

To conclude, we hope that through sharing our team's experience in this manual, we have impressed upon you, the mental health clinician, that working with functional seizures is an area of clinical practice that is interesting and

Referral triage by the mental health clinician (check that the following have been completed)

- A comprehensive medical assessment has been completed by a medical practitioner: physical examination, blood panel, and EEG (video EEG or EEG with review of video material by a paediatric neurologist).
- The medical practitioner has provided a positive diagnosis.
- The medical practitioner has provided an explanation.
- The young person and the family understand and accept the diagnosis.

Biopsychosocial assessment with the young person and the family

- The biopsychosocial assessment aims to bring to light the young person's developmental history in the context of the family story, including a timeline of physical, psychological, and relational stressors (the story of the family and the story of the symptoms).
- The biopsychosocial assessment allows the clinician, young person, and family to co-construct a formulation—a summary of predisposing, precipitating, and perpetuating factors.
- The formulation is used, in turn, to develop a treatment plan and to guide the treatment process.
- The young person and family need to understand the rationale for the treatment plan and to agree to (contract to) the treatment intervention (including the offered time frame).

Psychoeducation

- The initial psychoeducation intervention is delivered at the end of the biopsychosocial assessment. The clinician explains functional seizures again. The clinician also provides information about the treatment components and their rationale.
- Psychoeducation is usually repeated during, and integrated into, some of the early treatment sessions.

The mind-body treatment intervention with the mental health clinician and multidisciplinary team

Daily timetable	Five-Step Plan for Managing Functional Seizures	Daily pleasurable exercise or physiotherapy	Working with the family	Working with the school	Medications	Longer-term individual or family therapy
• Stabilise rhythms of daily living • Document daily practice of treatment elements	• Identify warning signs • Make yourself safe • Implement mind-body regulation strategy • Ride it out • Implement mind-body regulation strategy	• As a physical regulation strategy • To address deconditioning • To build resilience • For neuroprotection • To manage pain • To help sleep	• To address focus-of-attention • To hold positive expectations • To address family issues that contribute to the presentation	• Develop a school-based health care plan for managing functional seizures in the school setting • Implement integration of young person back to school	• To help decrease arousal • To help with sleep • For comorbid anxiety or depression • For comorbid functional gut disorders	• To work on issues not addressed by the Five-Step Plan intervention • To treat comorbid mental health disorders • To engage in a trauma-processing intervention • Ongoing family, parenting, or marital work (with parents)

Taking the mind-body intervention home

The family continues to implement all components of the mind-body intervention (as relevant to their particular context).

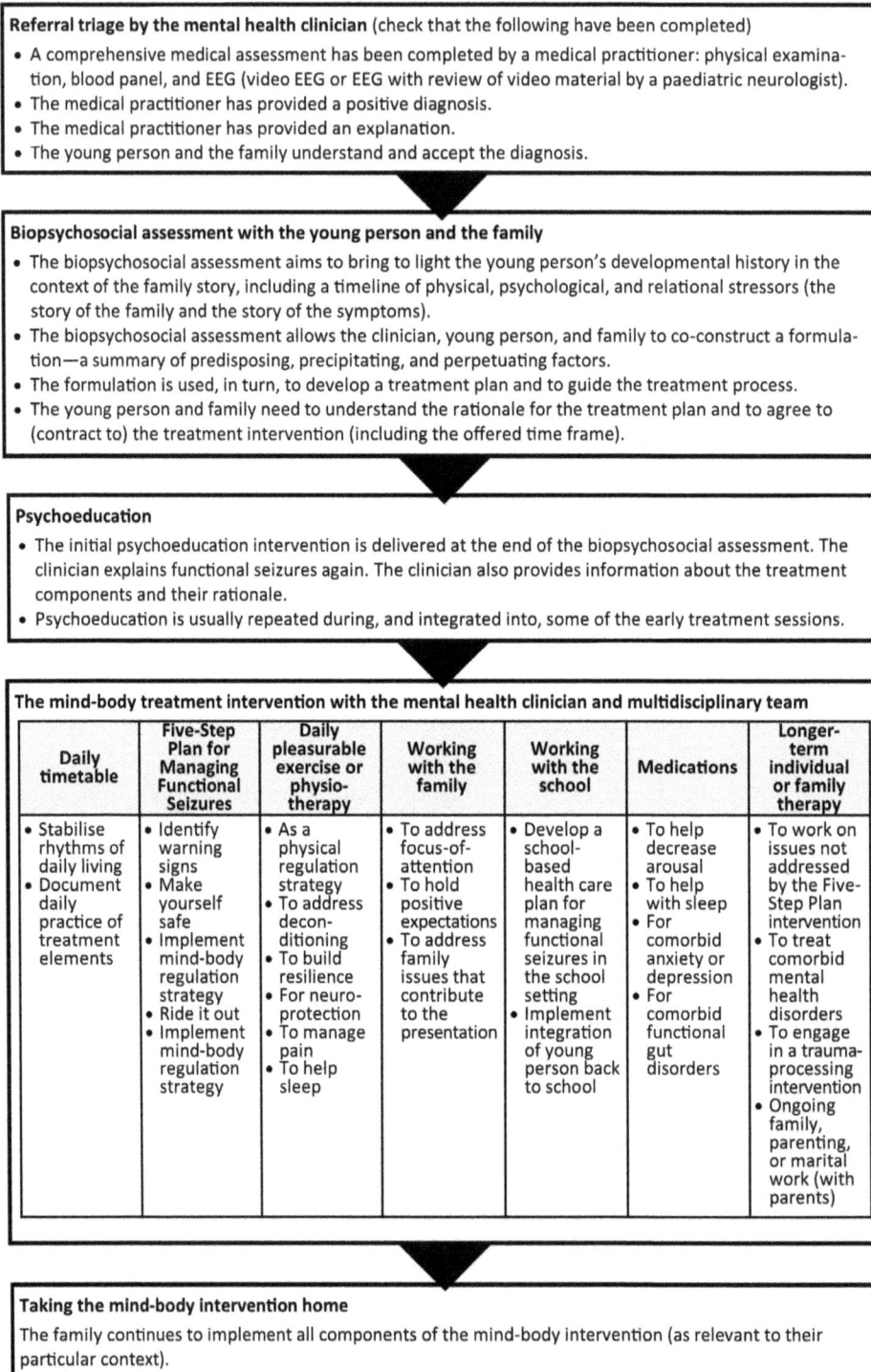

Figure 16.1 Flowchart of therapeutic process.
© Kasia Kozlowska and Blanche Savage 2022

rewarding. We hope that the manual answers questions, allays concerns, and highlights how you can use your existing skills — and build new skills — to help these young people and their families. We hope the manual provides a path forward, that it leads to improved care for this particular group of patients, and that it leads to a change in the broader culture of care.

References

Academy for Guided Imagery. (2022) *What is interactive guided imagery*. https://acadgi.com/about_sitemap/what_is_igi/

Akinsanya, A., Marwaha, R., & Tampi, R. R. (2017). Prazosin in children and adolescents with posttraumatic stress disorder who have nightmares: A systematic review. *J Clin Psychopharmacol, 37*(1), 84–88. https://doi.org/10.1097/JCP.0000000000000638

American Psychiatric Association. (2013). *Diagnostic and statistical manual of mental disorders* (5th ed.). https://doi.org/10.1176/appi.books.9780890425596

Arnold, M. M., Muller-Oerlinghausen, B., Hemrich, N., & Bonsch, D. (2020). Effects of psychoactive massage in outpatients with depressive disorders: A randomized controlled mixed-methods Study. *Brain Sci, 10*(10). https://doi.org/10.3390/brainsci10100676

Arnsten, A. F. (2009). Stress signalling pathways that impair prefrontal cortex structure and function. *Nat Rev Neurosci, 10*(6), 410–422. https://doi.org/10.1038/nrn2648

Arnsten, A. F. (2015). Stress weakens prefrontal networks: Molecular insults to higher cognition. *Nat Neurosci, 18*(10), 1376–1385. https://doi.org/10.1038/nn.4087

Arnsten, A. F., Raskind, M. A., Taylor, F. B., & Connor, D. F. (2015). The effects of stress exposure on prefrontal cortex: Translating basic research into successful treatments for post-traumatic stress disorder. *Neurobiol Stress, 1*, 89–99. https://doi.org/10.1016/j.ynstr.2014.10.002

Asadi-Pooya, A. A., Brigo, F., Kozlowska, K., Perez, D. L., Pretorius, C., Sawchuk, T., Saxena, A., Tolchin, B., & Valente, K. D. (2021). Social aspects of life in patients with functional seizures: Closing the gap in the biopsychosocial formulation. *Epilepsy Behav, 117*, 107903. https://doi.org/10.1016/j.yebeh.2021.107903

Baumgart, S. B., Baumbach-Kraft, A., & Lorenz, J. (2020). Effect of psycho-regulatory massage therapy on pain and depression in women with chronic and/or somatoform back pain: A randomized controlled trial. *Brain Sci, 10*(10), 721. https://doi.org/10.3390/brainsci10100721

Beck, A. T. (1976). *Cognitive therapy and the emotional disorders*. New American Library.

Benarroch, E. E. (2007). Brainstem respiratory chemosensitivity: New insights and clinical implications. *Neurology, 68*(24), 2140–2143. https://doi.org/10.1212/01.wnl.0000266560.60371.98

Benedetti, F. (2013). Placebo and the new physiology of the doctor-patient relationship. *Physiol Rev, 93*(3), 1207–1246. https://doi.org/10.1152/physrev.00043.2012

Blakeslee, A. (2021). *Bringing the body into therapy: Clinical tools from somatic experiencing* [digital seminar]. https://www.psychotherapy.com.au/item/bringing-body-therapy-clinical-tools-somatic-experiencing-89056

Bloch-Atefi, A., & Smith, J. (2015). The effectiveness of body-oriented psychotherapy: A review of the literature. *Psychother Couns J Aust, 3*(1).

Boyce, W. T., Levitt, P., Martinez, F. D., McEwen, B. S., & Shonkoff, J. P. (2021). Genes, environments, and time: The biology of adversity and resilience. *Pediatrics, 147*(2). https://doi.org/10.1542/peds.2020-1651

Braun, M., Sawchuk, T., Simpkins, A., Heer, N., Johnson, J., Esser, M., & Jacobs, J. (2021). *Quantitative EEG during hyperventilation as a biomarker for pediatric psychogenic non-epileptic seizures (PNES)*. Poster session presented at the annual meeting of the American Epilepsy Society, Chicago, USA.

Brown, L. A., Gaudiano, B. A., & Miller, I. W. (2011). Investigating the similarities and differences between practitioners of second- and third-wave cognitive-behavioral therapies. *Behav Modif, 35*(2), 187–200. https://doi.org/10.1177/0145445510393730

Brown, R. P., & Gerbarg, P. L. (2005). Sudarshan Kriya yogic breathing in the treatment of stress, anxiety, and depression: Part I—neurophysiologic model. *J Altern Complement Med, 11*(1), 189–201. https://doi.org/10.1089/acm.2005.11.189

Burridge, N., & Symons, K. (2018). *Australian don't rush to crush handbook* (3rd ed.). Society of Hospital Pharmacists of Australia.

Carson, A., Lehn, A., Ludwig, L., & Stone, J. (2015). Explaining functional disorders in the neurology clinic: A photo story. *Pract Neurol, 16*(1), 56–61. https://doi.org/10.1136/practneurol-2015-001242

Centre for Clinical Interventions. *Sleep hygiene.* https://www.cci.health.wa.gov.au/~/media/CCI/Mental-Health-Professionals/Sleep/Sleep—-Information-Sheets/Sleep-Information-Sheet—-04—-Sleep-Hygiene.pdf

Chandra, P., Kozlowska, K., Cruz, C., Baslet, G. C., Perez, D. L., & Garralda, M. E. (2017). Hyperventilation-induced non-epileptic seizures in an adolescent boy with pediatric medical traumatic stress. *Harv Rev Psychiatry*, *25*(4), 180–190. https://doi.org/10.1097/HRP.0000000000000131

Chrousos, G., Vgontzas, A. N., & Kritikou, I. (Updated 2020, November 24). HPA axis and sleep. In K. R. Feingold, B. Anawalt, & A. Boyce (Eds.), *Comprehensive FREE online endocrinology book*. Endotext [Internet]. https://www.ncbi.nlm.nih.gov/books/NBK279071/

Chrousos, G. P., Loriaux, D. L., & Gold, P. W. (1988). The concept of stress and its historical development. . In G. P. Chrousos, D. L. Loriaux, & P. W. Gold (Eds.), *Mechanisms of physical and emotional stress* (pp. 3–7). Plenum Press.

Chudleigh, C., Kozlowska, K., Kothur, K., Davies, F., Baxter, H., Landini, A., Hazell, P., & Baslet, G. (2013). Managing non-epileptic seizures and psychogenic dystonia in an adolescent girl with preterm brain injury. *Harv Rev Psychiatry*, *21*(3), 163–174. https://doi.org/10.1097/HRP.0b013e318293b29f

Chudleigh, C., Savage, B., Cruz, C., Lim, M., McClure, G., Palmer, D. M., Spooner, C. J., Kozlowska, K. (2019). Use of respiratory rates and heart rate variability in the assessment and treatment of children and adolescents with functional somatic symptoms. *Clin Child Psychol Psychiatry*, *24*(1), 29–39. https://doi.org/10.1177/1359104518807742

Chung, J., Mukerji, S., & Kozlowska, K. (2022). Cortisol and α-amylase awakening response in children and adolescents with functional neurological (conversion) disorder. *Aust N Z J Psychiatry*.

Cleveland Clinic (2021). *How box breathing can help you destress*. https://health.clevelandclinic.org/box-breathing-benefits/

Cohen, J. A., Mannarino, A. P., & Deblinger, E. (2012). *Trauma-focused CBT for children and adolescents: Treatment applications*. Guilford Press.

Craig, A. D. (2003a). Interoception: The sense of the physiological condition of the body. *Curr Opin Neurobiol*, *13*(4), 500–505. https://doi.org/10.1016/S0959-4388(03)00090-4

Craig, A. D. (2003b). A new view of pain as a homeostatic emotion. *Trends Neurosci*, *26*(6), 303–307. https://doi.org/10.1016/S0166-2236(03)00123-1

Cristea, I. A., Vecchi, T., & Cuijpers, P. (2021). Top-down and bottom-up pathways to developing psychological interventions. *JAMA Psychiatry*, *78*(6), 593–594. https://doi.org/10.1001/jamapsychiatry.2020.4793

Crittenden, P. M., & Landini, A. (2011). *Assessing adult attachment: A dynamic-maturational approach to discourse analysis*. Norton.

Damasio, A., & Carvalho, G. B. (2013). The nature of feelings: Evolutionary and neurobiological origins. *Nat Rev Neurosci*, *14*(2), 143–152. https://doi.org/10.1038/nrn3403

Damasio, A. R. (1994). *Descartes' error: Emotion, reason, and the human brain*. G. P. Putnam.

Damasio, A. R. (2018). *The strange order of things: Life, feeling, and the making of cultures*. Pantheon Books.

Duraccio, K. M., Whitacre, C., Krietsch, K. N., Zhang, N., Summer, S., Price, M., Saelens, B. E., & Beebe, D. W. (2022). Losing sleep by staying up late leads adolescents to consume more carbohydrates and a higher glycemic load. *Sleep*, *45*(3). https://doi.org/10.1093/sleep/zsab269

Edwards, M. J., Adams, R. A., Brown, H., Parees, I., & Friston, K. J. (2012). A Bayesian account of 'hysteria'. *Brain*, *135*(Pt 11), 3495–3512. https://doi.org/10.1093/brain/aws129

Engel, G. L., Ferris, E. B., & Logan, M. (1947). Hyperventilation: Analysis of clinical symptomatology. *Ann Intern Med*, *27*(5), 683–704.

Erickson, M. H. (1982). My voice will go with you: The teaching teaching tales of Milton H. Erickson. Norton.

Erickson, M. H. (1954). Pseudo-orientation in time as a hypnotherapeutic procedure. *J Clin Exp Hypn*, *2*(4), 261–283.

Ernsberger, P., & Haxhiu, M. A. (1997). The I1-imidazoline-binding site is a functional receptor mediating vasodepression via the ventral medulla. *Am J Physiol*, *273*(5), R1572–1579. https://doi.org/10.1152/ajpregu.1997.273.5.R1572

Farnfield, S., Hautamaki, A., Nørbech, P., & Sahar, N. (2010). DMM assessments of attachment and adaptation: Procedures, validity and utility. *Clin Child Psychol Psychiatry*, *15*(3), 313–328.

Filaire, E., Ferreira, J. P., Oliveira, M., & Massart, A. (2013). Diurnal patterns of salivary alpha-amylase and cortisol secretion in female adolescent tennis players after 16 weeks of training. *Psychoneuroendocrinology*, *38*(7), 1122–1132. https://doi.org/10.1016/j.psyneuen.2012.11.001

Fleming, S., Thompson, M., Stevens, R., Heneghan, C., Pluddemann, A., Maconochie, I., Tarassenko, L., & Mant, D. (2011). Normal ranges of heart rate and respiratory rate in children from birth to 18 years of age: A systematic review of observational studies. *Lancet*, *377*(9770), 1011–1018. https://doi.org/10.1016/S0140-6736(10)62226-X

Førdea, S., Breen Hernera, L., Helland, I. B., & Diseth, T. H. (forthcoming). The biopsychosocial model in paediatric clinical practice: A multidisciplinary approach to somatic symptom disorders. *Acta Paediatr*, *111*(11), 2115–2124. https://doi.org/10.1111/apa.16517

Fobian, A. D., Long, D. M., & Szaflarski, J. P. (2020). Retraining and control therapy for pediatric psychogenic non-epileptic seizures. *Ann Clin Transl Neurol*, *7*(8), 1410–1419. https://doi.org/10.1002/acn3.51138

Gelder, M. G. (1997). The scientific foundations of cognitive behaviour therapy. In D. M. Clark & C. G. Fairburn (Eds.), *The science and practice of cognitive behaviour therapy* (pp. 27–46). Oxford University Press.

Gerritsen, R. J. S., & Band, G. P. H. (2018). Breath of life: The respiratory vagal stimulation model of contemplative activity. *Front Hum Neurosci*, *12*, 397. https://doi.org/10.3389/fnhum.2018.00397

Gianaros, P. J., & Wager, T. D. (2015). Brain-body pathways linking psychological stress and physical health. *Curr Dir Psychol Sci*, *24*(4), 313–321. https://doi.org/10.1177/0963721415581476

Gordon, C., Riess, H., & Waldinger, R. J. (2005). The formulation as a collaborative conversation. *Harv Rev Psychiatry*, *13*(2), 112–123. https://doi.org/10.1080/10673220590956519

Gray, N., Savage, B., Scher, S., & Kozlowska, K. (2020). Psychologically informed physical therapy for children and adolescents with functional neurological symptoms: The Wellness Approach. *J Neuropsychiatry Clin Neurosci*, *32*(4), 389–395. https://doi.org/10.1176/appi.neuropsych.19120355

Guendelman, S., Medeiros, S., & Rampes, H. (2017). Mindfulness and emotion regulation: Insights from neurobiological, psychological, and clinical studies. *Front Psychol*, *8*, 220. https://doi.org/10.3389/fpsyg.2017.00220

Good Therapy. (2022). *Guided therapeutic imagery*. https://www.goodtherapy.org/learn-about-therapy/types/guided-therapeutic-imagery

Gumbiner, C. H. (2003). Precordial catch syndrome. *South Med J*, *96*(1), 38–41. https://www.ncbi.nlm.nih.gov/pubmed/12602711

Haley, J. (1973). *Uncommon therapy: The psychiatric techniques of Milton H. Erickson, M.D.* Norton.

Han, V. X., Kozlowska, K., Kothur, K., Lorentzos, M., Wong, W. K., Mohammad, S. S., Savage, B., Chudleigh, C., & Dale, R. C. (2022). Rapid onset functional tic-like behaviours in children and adolescents during COVID-19: Clinical features, assessment and biopsychosocial treatment approach. *J Paediatr Child Health*. https://doi.org/10.1111/jpc.15932

Harris, R., & Hayes, S. C. (2007). *The happiness trap: Stop struggling, start living*. Exisle Publishing.

Hayes, S. C. (2004). Acceptance and commitment therapy, relational frame theory, and the third wave of behavioral and cognitive therapies. *Behav Ther, 35*(4), 639–665.

Hayes, S. C., & Hofmann, S. G. (2017). The third wave of cognitive behavioral therapy and the rise of process-based care. *World Psychiatry, 16*(3), 245–246. https://doi.org/10.1002/wps.20442

Hayes, S. C., & Hofmann, S. G. (2018). *Process-based CBT: The science and core clinical competencies of cognitive behavioral therapy.* Context Press.

Healing Waterfall. *History of guided imagery.* (2013). http://guidedimagery-downloads.com/history-of-guided-imagery/

Helgeland, H., Savage, B., & Kozlowska, K. (forthcoming). Hypnosis in the treatment of functional somatic symptoms in children and adolescents. In. J. H. Linden, G. De Benedittis, L. I. Sugarman, & K. Varga (Eds.). *Routledge International Handbook of Clinical Hypnosis.* Routledge.

Helgeland, H., Gjone, H., & Diseth, T. H. (2022). The biopsychosocial board — a conversation tool for broad diagnostic assessment and identification of effective treatment of children with functional somatic disorders. *Hum Syst, 2*(3), 144–157.

Helgeland, H., Lindheim, M. Ø., Diseth, T. H., & Brodal, P. A. (2021). Clinical hypnosis — a revitalisation of the art of medicine. *Tidsskr Nor Laegeforen, 141*(7). https:10.4045/tidsskr.21.0098

Henderson, S., & Martin, A. (2014). Case formulation and integration of information in child and adolescent mental health. In J. M. Rey (Ed.), *IACAPAP e-textbook of child and adolescent mental health.* International Association for Child and Adolescent Psychiatry and Allied Professions.

Hetrick, S. E., McKenzie, J. E., Bailey, A. P., Sharma, V., Moller, C. I., Badcock, P. B., Cox, G. R., Merry, Sally N., & Meader, N. (2021). New generation antidepressants for depression in children and adolescents: A network meta-analysis. *Cochrane Database Syst Rev, 5*, CD013674. https://doi.org/10.1002/14651858.CD013674.pub2

Heyman, I., Liang, H., & Hedderly, T. (2021). COVID-19 related increase in childhood tics and tic-like attacks. *Arch Dis Child.* https://doi.org/10.1136/archdischild-2021-321748

Hummel, K. V., Trautmann, S., Venz, J., Thomas, S., & Schafer, J. (2021). Repetitive negative thinking: Transdiagnostic correlate and risk factor for mental disorders? A proof-of-concept study in German soldiers before and after deployment to Afghanistan. *BMC Psychol, 9*(1), 198. https://doi.org/10.1186/s40359-021-00696-2

Huss, M., Chen, W., & Ludolph, A. G. (2016). Guanfacine extended release: A new pharmacological treatment option in Europe. *Clin Drug Investig,* *36*(1), 1–25. https://doi.org/10.1007/s40261-015-0336-0

Hyams, J. S., Di Lorenzo, C., Saps, M., Shulman, R. J., Staiano, A., & van Tilburg, M. (2016). Functional disorders: Children and adolescents. *Gastroenterology.* https://doi.org/10.1053/j.gastro.2016.02.015

James, W. (1890). *The principles of psychology. Vol. 1.* Henry Holt.

Jungilligens, J., Paredes-Echeverri, S., Popkirov, S., Barrett, L. F., & Perez, D. L. (2022). A new science of emotion: Implications for functional neurological disorder. *Brain, 145*(8), 2648–2663. https://doi.org/10.1093/brain/awac204

Kabat-Zinn, J. (1982). An outpatient program in behavioral medicine for chronic pain patients based on the practice of mindfulness meditation: Theoretical considerations and preliminary results. *Gen Hosp Psychiatry, 4*(1), 33–47. https://doi.org/10.1016/0163-8343(82)90026-3

Kabat-Zinn, J. (2003). Mindfulness-based interventions in context: Past, present, and future. *Clin Psychol, 10*(4), 144–156. https://doi.org/10.1093/clipsy.bpg016

Kain, K. L., & Terrell, S. J. (2018). *Nurturing resilience: Helping clients move forward from developmental trauma: An integrative somatic approach.* North Atlantic Books.

Khachane, Y., Kozlowska, K., Savage, B., McClure, G., Butler, G., Gray, N., Worth, A., Mihailovich, S., Perez, D., Helgeland, H., & Chrousos, G. P. (2019). Twisted in pain: The multidisciplinary treatment approach to functional dystonia. *Harv Rev Psychiatry, 27*(6), 359–381. https://doi.org/10.1097/HRP.0000000000000237

Kim, Y.-N., Gray, N., Jones, A., Scher, S., & Kozlowska, K. (2021). The role of physiotherapy in the management of functional neurological disorder in children and adolescents. *Semin Pediatr Neurol,* 100947. https://doi.org/10.1016/j.spen.2021.100947

Kleckner, I. R., Zhang, J., Touroutoglou, A., Chanes, L., Xia, C., Simmons, W. K., . . . Barrett, L. F. (2017). Evidence for a large-scale brain system supporting allostasis and interoception in humans. *Nat Hum Behav, 1,* 0069. https://doi.org/10.1038/s41562-017-0069

Kohen, D. P., & Kaiser, P. (2014). Clinical hypnosis with children and adolescents—What? Why? How?: Origins, applications, and efficacy. *Children (Basel), 1*(2), 74–98. https://doi.org/10.3390/children1020074

Kozlowska, K. (2013). Stress, distress, and bodytalk: Co-constructing formulations with patients who present with somatic symptoms. *Harv Rev Psychiatry, 21*(6), 314–333. https://doi.org/10.1097/HRP.0000000000000008

Kozlowska, K., Brown, K. J., Palmer, D. M., & Williams, L. M. (2013). Specific biases for identifying facial expression of emotion in children and adolescents with conversion disorders. *Psychosom Med*, *75*(3), 272–280. https://doi.org/10.1097/PSY.0b013e318286be43

Kozlowska, K., Chudleigh, C., Elliott, B., & Landini, A. (2016). The body comes to family therapy: Treatment of a school-aged boy with hyperventilation-induced non-epileptic seizures. *Clin Child Psychol Psychiatry*, *21*(4), 669–685. https://doi.org/10.1177/1359104515621960

Kozlowska, K., Gray, N., Scher, S., & Savage, B. (2020). Psychologically informed physiotherapy as part of a multidisciplinary rehabilitation program for children and adolescents with functional neurological disorder: Physical and mental health outcomes. *J Paediatr Child Health*, *57*(1), 73–79. https://doi.org/doi:10.1111/jpc.15122

Kozlowska, K., Griffiths, K. R., Foster, S. L., Linton, J., Williams, L. M., & Korgaonkar, M. S. (2017). Grey matter abnormalities in children and adolescents with functional neurological symptom disorder. *Neuroimage Clin*, *15*, 306–314. https://doi.org/10.1016/j.nicl.2017.04.028

Kozlowska, K., Melkonian, D., Spooner, C. J., Scher, S., & Meares, R. (2017). Cortical arousal in children and adolescents with functional neurological symptoms during the auditory oddball task. *Neuroimage Clin*, *13*, 228–236. https://doi.org/10.1016/j.nicl.2016.10.016

Kozlowska, K., & Mohammad, S. (forthcoming). Functional neurological disorder in children and adolescents: Assessment and treatment. In L. Sivaswamy & D. Kamat (Eds.), *Symptom-Based Approach to Pediatric Neurology*. Springer Nature.

Kozlowska, K., Palmer, D. M., Brown, K. J., McLean, L., Scher, S., Gevirtz, R., Chudleigh, C. & Williams, L. M. (2015). Reduction of autonomic regulation in children and adolescents with conversion disorders. *Psychosom Med*, *77*(4), 356–370. https://doi.org/10.1097/PSY.0000000000000184

Kozlowska, K., Rampersad, R., Cruz, C., Shah, U., Chudleigh, C., Soe, S., Gill, D., Scher, S., & Carrive, P. (2017). The respiratory control of carbon dioxide in children and adolescents referred for treatment of psychogenic non-epileptic seizures. *Eur Child Adolesc Psychiatry*, *26*(10), 1207–1217. https://doi.org/10.1007/s00787-017-0976-0

Kozlowska, K., Sawchuk, T., Waugh, J. L., Helgeland, H., Baker, J., Scher, S., & Fobian, A. (2021). Changing the culture of care for children and adolescents with functional neurological disorder. *Epilepsy Behav Rep*, *16*, 1004486. https://doi.org/10.1016/j.ebr.2021.100486

Kozlowska, K., Scher, S., & Helgeland, H. (2020). *Functional somatic symptoms in children and adolescents: A stress-system approach to assessment and treatment.* Palgrave Macmillan.

Kozlowska, K., Scher, S., & Williams, L. M. (2011). Patterns of emotional-cognitive functioning in pediatric conversion patients: Implications for the conceptualization of conversion disorders. *Psychosom Med, 73*(9), 775–788. https://doi.org/10.1097/PSY.0b013e3182361e12

Kozlowska, K., Walker, P., McLean, L., & Carrive, P. (2015). Fear and the defense cascade: Clinical implications and management. *Harv Rev Psychiatry, 23*(4), 263–287. https://doi.org/10.1097/HRP.0000000000000065

Kumarah Yoga. (2022). *How to make a mindfulness glitter calm down jar.* https://kumarahyoga.com/how-to-make-a-mindfulness-glitter-calm-down-jar/

Lamotte, G., Shouman, K., & Benarroch, E. E. (2021). Stress and central autonomic network. *Auton Neurosci, 235,* 102870. https://doi.org/10.1016/j.autneu.2021.102870

Lappin, J. (1988). Family therapy: A structural approach. In R. A. Dorfman (Ed.), *Paradigms of clinical social work* (pp. 220–252). Brunner/Mazel.

Levine, P. A. (2010). *In an unspoken voice: How the body releases trauma and restores goodness.* North Atlantic Books.

Li, Y., Hao, Y., Fan, F., & Zhang, B. (2018). The role of microbiome in insomnia, circadian disturbance and depression. *Front Psychiatry, 9,* 669. https://doi.org/10.3389/fpsyt.2018.00669

Linehan, M. M. (2018). *Cognitive-behavioral treatment of borderline personality disorder.* Guilford Press.

MacKinnon, L. (2014). Deactivating the buttons: Integrating radical exposure tapping with a family therapy framework. *Aust N Z J Fam Ther, 35*(3), 244–260. https://doi.org/10.1002/anzf.1070

McCraty, R., & Childre, D. (2010). Coherence: Bridging personal, social, and global health. *Altern Ther Health Med, 16*(4), 10–24. http://www.ncbi.nlm.nih.gov/pubmed/20653292

Minuchin, S. (1974). *Families and family therapy.* Harvard University Press.

Nelson, C. A. (2013). Biological embedding of early life adversity. *JAMA Pediatr, 167*(12), 1098–1100. https://doi.org/10.1001/jamapediatrics.2013.3768

Norman, L., Lawrence, N., Iles, A., Benattayallah, A., & Karl, A. (2015). Attachment-security priming attenuates amygdala activation to social and linguistic threat. *Soc Cogn Affect Neurosci, 10*(6), 832–839. https://doi.org/10.1093/scan/nsu127

Norman Wells, J., Skowron, E. A., Scholtes, C. M., & DeGarmo, D. S. (2020). Differential physiological sensitivity to child compliance behaviors in abusing, neglectful, and non-maltreating mothers. *Dev Psychopathol, 32*(2), 531–543. https://doi.org/10.1017/S0954579419000270

Nunn, K. (1998). Neuropsychiatry in childhood: Residential treatment. In J. Green & B. Jacobs (Eds.), *In-patient child psychiatry: Modern practice, research and the future* (pp. 259–283). Routledge.

Ogden, P., & Fisher, J. (2015). *Sensorimotor psychotherapy: Interventions for trauma and attachment.* Norton.

Pace-Schott, E. F., Amole, M. C., Aue, T., Balconi, M., Bylsma, L. M., Critchley, H., Demaree, H. A., Friedman, B. H., Gooding, A. E. K., Gosseries, O., Jovanovic T., Kirby, L. A., Kozlowska, K., Laureys, S., Lowe, L. Magee, K., Marin, M-F., Merner, A. R., Robinson, J. L., Smith, R. C., VanElzakker, M. B. (2019). Physiological feelings. *Neurosci Biobehav Rev., 103,* 267–304. https://doi.org/10.1016/j.neubiorev.2019.05.002

Pagani, M., Di Lorenzo, G., Monaco, L., Daverio, A., Giannoudas, I., La Porta, P., Verardo, A. R., Niolu, C., Fernandez, I., & Siracusano, A. (2015). Neurobiological response to EMDR therapy in clients with different psychological traumas. *Front Psychol, 6,* 1614. https://doi.org/10.3389/fpsyg.2015.01614

Payne, P., Levine, P. A., & Crane-Godreau, M. A. (2015). Somatic experiencing: Using interoception and proprioception as core elements of trauma therapy. *Front Psychol, 6,* 93. https://doi.org/10.3389/fpsyg.2015.00093

Pesheva, E. (2021, November 16). *Diet, gut microbes,and immunity. Research in mice shows how diet alters immune system function through a gutmicrobe.* Harvard Medical School. News and Research. https://hms.harvard.edu/news/diet-gut-microbes-immunity

Perez, D. L., Edwards, M. J., Nielsen, G., Kozlowska, K., Hallett, M., & LaFrance, W. C., Jr. (2021). Decade of progress in motor functional neurological disorder: continuing the momentum. *J Neurol Neurosurg Psychiatry, 16,* 668–677. https://doi.org/10.1136/jnnp-2020-323953

Porges, S. W. (2009). The polyvagal theory: New insights into adaptive reactions of the autonomic nervous system. *Cleve Clin J Med, 76 Suppl 2,* S86–90. https://doi.org/10.3949/ccjm.76.s2.17

Porges, S. W. (2018). *Methods and systems for reducing sound sensitivities and improving auditory processing, behavioral state regulation and social engagement behaviors* (U.S. patent No. 10,029,068 B2). U.S. Patent and Trade-mark Office. http://patft.uspto.gov/netacgi/nph-Parser?patent-number=10029068 B2

Pringsheim, T., Ganos, C., McGuire, J. F., Hedderly, T., Woods, D., Gilbert, D. L., Piacentini, J., Dale, R.C., & Martino, D. (2021). Rapid onset functional tic-like behaviors in young females during the COVID-19 pandemic. *Mov Disord, 36*(12), 2707–2713. https://doi.org/10.1002/mds.28778

Rhodes, A. W. P. (2011). *A practical guide to family therapy: Structured guidelines and key skills.* IP Communications.

Radmanesh, M., Jalili, M., & Kozlowska, K. (2020). Activation of functional brain networks in children and adolescents with psychogenic non-epileptic seizures. *Front Hum Neurosci, 14*, 339. https://doi.org/https://doi.org/10.3389/fnhum.2020.00339

Rajabalee, N., Kozlowska, K., Lee, S. Y., Savage, B., Hawkes, C., Siciliano, D., Porges, S. W., Pick, S., & Torbey, S. (2022). Neuromodulation using computer altered music to treat a ten-year-old child unresponsive to standard interventions for functional neurological disorder. *Harv Rev Psychiatry, 30*(5):303–316. https://doi.org/10.1097/HRP.0000000000000341

Rapee, R., Wignall, A., Spence, S., Cobham, V., & Lyneham, H. (2008). *Helping your anxious child: A step by step guide for parents.* (2nd ed.). New Harbinger.

Rai, S., Foster, S., Griffiths, K. R., Breukelaar, I. A., Kozlowska, K., & Korgaonkar, M. S. (2022). Altered resting-state neural networks in children and adolescents with functional neurological disorder. *Neuroimage Clin, 35*, 103110. https://doi.org/10.1016/j.nicl.2022.103110

Rask, C. U., Ornbol, E., Olsen, E. M., Fink, P., & Skovgaard, A. M. (2013). Infant behaviors are predictive of functional somatic symptoms at ages 5–7 years: Results from the Copenhagen Child Cohort CCC2000. *J Pediatr, 162*, 335–342. https://doi.org/10.1016/j.jpeds.2012.08.001

Rathus, J. H., & Miller, A. L. (2002). Dialectical behavior therapy adapted for suicidal adolescents. *Suicide Life Threat Behav, 32*(2), 146–157. http://www.ncbi.nlm.nih.gov/pubmed/12079031

Ratnamohan, L., MacKinnon, L., Lim, M., Webster, R., Waters, K., Kozlowska, K., Silberg, J., Greenwald, R., & Ribeiro, M. (2018). Ambushed by memories of trauma: Memory-processing interventions in an adolescent boy with nocturnal dissociative episodes. *Harv Rev Psychiatry, 26*(4), 228–236. https://doi.org/10.1097/HRP.0000000000000195

Rhodes, P., & Wallis, A. (2011). A practical guide to family therapy: Structured guidelines and key skills. IP Communications.

Rizvi, S. L. (2019). *Chain analysis in dialectical behavior therapy*. Guilford Press.

Rosenwinkel, E. T., Bloomfield, D. M., Arwady, M. A., & Goldsmith, R. L. (2001). Exercise and autonomic function in health and cardiovascular disease. *Cardiol Clin*, *19*(3), 369–387. https://doi.org/10.1016/s0733-8651(05)70223-x

Rowe, P. C. (2014). *General information brochure on orthostatic intolerance and its treatment.* http://www.dysautonomiainternational.org/pdf/RoweOIsummary.pdf

Saarman, E. (2006). *Feeling the beat: Symposium explores the therapeutic effects of rhythmic music.* https://news.stanford.edu/news/2006/may31/brainwave-053106.html

Salford Royal NHS Foundation Trust. (2021). *Understanding functional neurological disorder.* https://gmisdn.org.uk/wp-content/uploads/2020/05/Understanding-FND-leaflet.pdf

Sawchuk, T., Buchhalter, J., & Senft, B. (2020a). Psychogenic nonepileptic seizures in children — prospective validation of a clinical care pathway & risk factors for treatment outcome. *Epilepsy Behav*, *105*, 106971. https://doi.org/10.1016/j.yebeh.2020.106971

Sawchuk, T., Buchhalter, J., & Senft, B. (2020b). Psychogenic non-epileptic seizures in children — psychophysiology & dissociative characteristics. *Psychiatry Res*, *294*, 113544. https://doi.org/10.1016/j.psychres.2020.113544

Scheffer, D. D. L., & Latini, A. (2020). Exercise-induced immune system response: Anti-inflammatory status on peripheral and central organs. *Biochim Biophys Acta Mol Basis Dis*, *1866*(10), 165823. https://doi.org/10.1016/j.bbadis.2020.165823

Schwartz, T. L., & Goradia, V. (2013). Managing insomnia: An overview of insomnia and pharmacologic treatment strategies in use and on the horizon. *Drugs Context*, *2013*, 212257. https://doi.org/10.7573/dic.212257

Shafir, T. (2016). Using movement to regulate emotion: Neurophysiological findings and their application in psychotherapy. *Front Psychol*, *7*, 1451. https://doi.org/10.3389/fpsyg.2016.01451

Shakeshaft, J. (2020). *6 breathing exercises that can help you relax in 10 minutes or less*. https://greatist.com/happiness/breathing-exercises-relax#Bottom-line

Sharma, A. A., & Szaflarski, J. P. (2021). Neuroinflammation as a pathophysiological factor in the development and maintenance of functional seizures: A hypothesis. *Epilepsy Behav Rep, 16,* 100496. https://doi.org/10.1016/j.ebr.2021.100496

Siegel, D. J. (1999). *The developing mind: How relationships and the brain interact to shape who we are.* Guilford Press.

Stahl, S. M. (2021). *Essential psychopharmacology: Neuroscientific basis and practical applications* (5th ed.). Cambridge University Press.

Stoddard, J. A., Afari, N., & Hayes, S. C. (2014). *The big book of act metaphors: A practitioner's guide to experiential exercises and metaphors in acceptance and commitment therapy.* New Harbinger Publications.

Tatum, W. O., Mani, J., Jin, K., Halford, J. J., Gloss, D., Fahoum, F., Maillard, L., Mothersill, I., & Beniczky, S. (2022). Minimum standards for inpatient long-term video-electroencephalographic monitoring: A clinical practice guideline of the International League Against Epilepsy and International Federation of Clinical Neurophysiology. *Epilepsia, 63*(2), 290–315. https://doi.org/10.1111/epi.16977

Thwaites, R., & Freeston, M. H. (2005). Safety-seeking behaviours: Fact or function? How can we clinically differentiate between safety behaviours and adaptive coping strategies across anxiety disorders? *Behav Cogn Psychother, 33,* 177–188. https://doi.org/10.1017/S1352465804001985

Tornblom, H., & Drossman, D. A. (2018). Psychotropics, antidepressants, and visceral analgesics in functional gastrointestinal disorders. *Curr Gastroenterol Rep, 20*(12), 58. https://doi.org/10.1007/s11894-018-0664-3

University of Nevada, Reno, Counseling Services. (n.d.). *Releasing stress through the power of music.* https://www.unr.edu/counseling/virtual-relaxation-room/releasing-stress-through-the-power-of-music

University of Wisconsin Stevens Point, University Health Service. (2005). *Precordial catch syndrome.* https://www.uwsp.edu/stuhealth/Documents/Other/Precordial%20Catch.pdf

van der Zalm, T., Alsma, J., van de Poll, S. W. E., Wessels, M. W., Riksen, N. P., & Versmissen, J. (2019). Postural orthostatic tachycardia syndrome (POTS): A common but unfamiliar syndrome. *Neth J Med, 77*(1), 3–9. https://www.ncbi.nlm.nih.gov/pubmed/30774097

Vassilopoulos, A., Mohammad, S., Dure, L., Kozlowska, K., & Fobian, A. D. (2022). Treatment approaches for functional neurologic disorders in children. *Curr Treat Options in Neurol, 24*(2), 77–97. https://doi.org/10.1007/s11940-022-00708-5

Vuilleumier, P., & Trost, W. (2015). Music and emotions: From enchantment to entrainment. *Ann N Y Acad Sci, 1337*, 212–222. https://doi.org/10.1111/nyas.12676

Wager, T. D., & Atlas, L. Y. (2015). The neuroscience of placebo effects: Connecting context, learning and health. *Nat Rev Neurosci, 16*(7), 403–418. https://doi.org/10.1038/nrn3976

Wallis, L. A., Healy, M., Undy, M. B., & Maconochie, I. (2005). Age related reference ranges for respiration rate and heart rate from 4 to 16 years. *Arch Dis Child, 90*(11), 1117–1121. https://doi.org/10.1136/adc.2004.068718

Wardrope, A., Dworetzky, B. A., Barkley, G. L., Baslet, G., Buchhalter, J., Doss, J., Goldstein, L. H., Hallett, M., Kozlowska, K., LaFrance, W. C., Jr., McGonigal, A., Mildon, B., Oto, M., Perez, D. L., Riker, E., Roberts, N. A., Stone, J., Tolchin, B., & Reuber, M. (2021). How to do things with words: Two seminars on the naming of functional (psychogenic, non-epileptic, dissociative, conversion, ...) seizures. *Seizure, 93*, 102–110. https://doi.org/10.1016/j.seizure.2021.10.016

Wells, R., Spurrier, A. J., Linz, D., Gallagher, C., Mahajan, R., Sanders, P., Page, A., & Lau, D. H. (2018). Postural tachycardia syndrome: Current perspectives. *Vasc Health Risk Manag, 14*, 1–11. https://doi.org/10.2147/VHRM.S127393

Whitehead, K., Kane, N., Wardrope, A., Kandler, R., & Reuber, M. (2017). Proposal for best practice in the use of video-EEG when psychogenic non-epileptic seizures are a possible diagnosis. *Clin Neurophysiol Pract, 2*, 130–139. https://doi.org/10.1016/j.cnp.2017.06.002

Wilson, L. D., Leath, T. C., & Patel, M. B. (2017). Management of paroxysmal sympathetic hyperactivity after traumatic brain injury. In K. Heidenreich (Ed.), *New therapeutics for traumatic brain injury: Prevention of secondary brain damage and enhancement of repair and regeneration* (pp. 145–158). Academic Press.

Winters, N. C., Hanson, G., & Stoyanova, V. (2007). The case formulation in child and adolescent psychiatry. *Child Adolesc Psychiatr Clin N Am, 16*(1), 111–132. https://doi.org/10.1016/j.chc.2006.07.010

Brief Summary of Research Findings That Underpin Our Current Understanding of Young People with Functional Seizures

An important theme that runs through the research about young people with functional neurological disorder (FND, including functional seizures) is the theme of regulation: the connection between functional neurological symptoms and the individual's capacity to regulate.

Regulation as a Developmental Process Shaped by the Attachment Figure

Regulation is a developmental process — a key developmental milestone of infancy, the preschool years, the school-age years, and adolescence. Regulation occurs as a series of stepping stones. See Figure A.1.

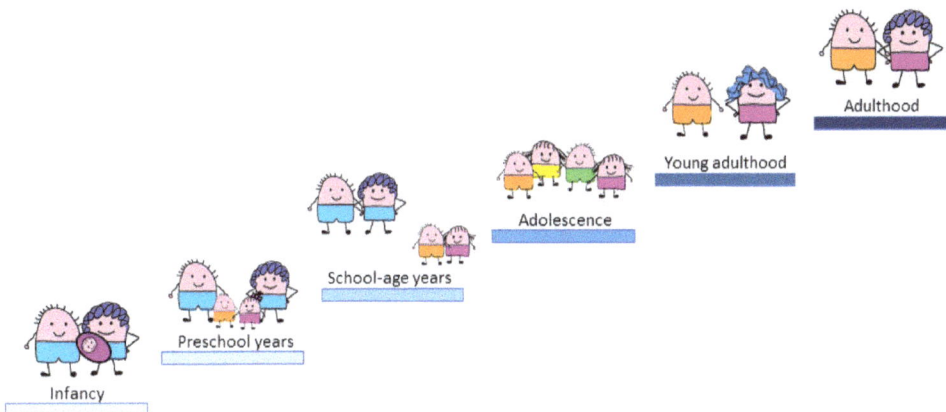

Figure A.1 Stages of development. Regulation is a developmental process — a series of stages. © Kasia Kozlowska 2021

In infancy, regulation is shaped by the attachment figure. It involves the establishment of sleep routines, feeding routines, capacity to settle (via the attachment figure's voice, facial expression, touch, and movement [rocking]).

When this stepping stone is compromised — that is, when the infant has problems with feeding, sleep, settling, or tactile reactivity — the risk of functional somatic symptoms later in childhood increases (Rask et al., 2013).

In the preschool years, regulation is a dyadic process. It involves co-regulation on the neurophysiological level — the autonomic nervous system, hypothalamic-pituitary-adrenal (HPA) axis, brain stress systems, and so on (Norman et al., 2015; Norman Wells et al., 2020). See Figure A.2.

When the child becomes upset or distressed — and the child's neurophysiological systems activate — the attachment figure helps the child down-regulate back to baseline (via voice, facial expression, touch, and movement).

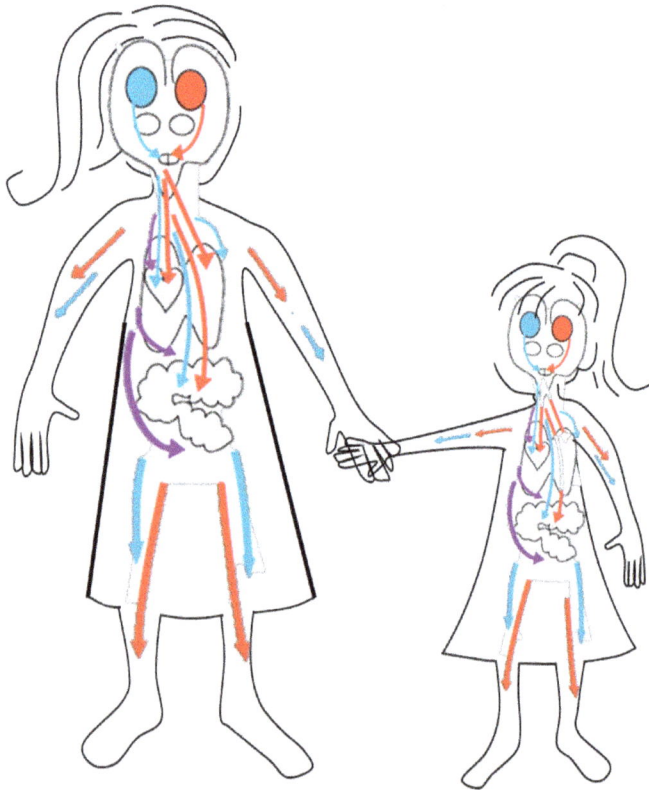

Figure A.2 Regulation as a dyadic process. Visual representation of co-regulation on the neurophysiological level, in this case pertaining to the autonomic nervous system. © Kasia Kozlowska 2019

Attachment research assesses the quality of these dyadic processes, including the child's capacity to regulate in the face of stress when an attachment figure is present.

Attachment in Young People with FND

A study from our Mind-Body Program comparing 76 children and adolescents with FND (aged 6–18 years) and healthy controls used structured interviews from the Dynamic Maturational Model of Attachment and Adaptation (DMM) to assess patterns of attachment (Kozlowska et al., 2011). Children and adolescents with functional seizures made up almost half the sample (36/76; 47%). As shown in Figure A.3, healthy controls (green dots) were classified into the normative patterns of attachment, and children with FND (red dots) were classified into the at-risk patterns of attachment. Twelve per cent of controls versus 75% of the children and adolescents with FND had unresolved loss and trauma. The findings from the study suggest, regarding the latter group, a long-standing history of relational stress and a chronic disruption of what are normally comfortable and nurturing attachments.

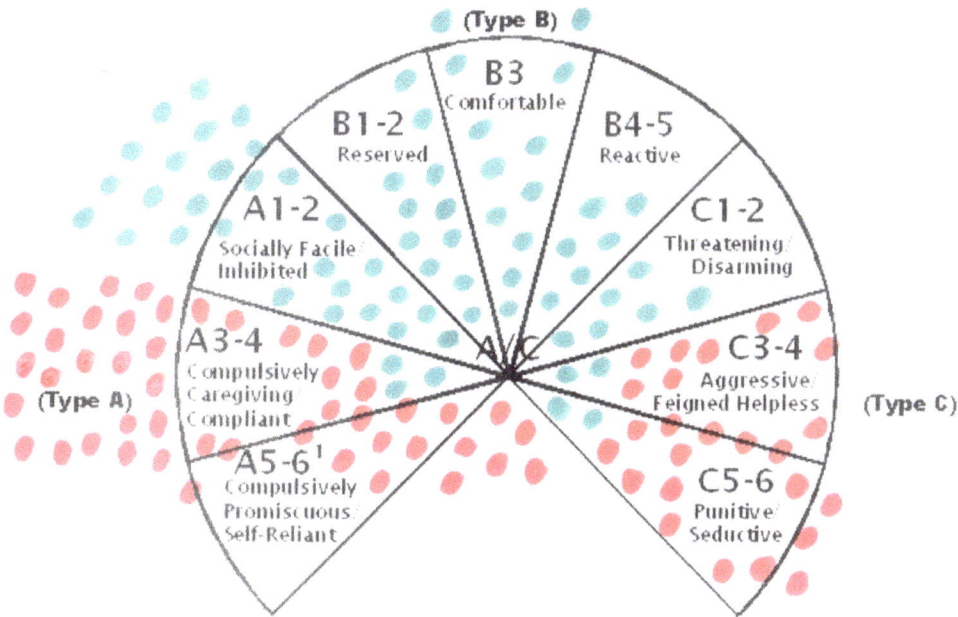

Figure A.3 Patterns of attachment in children with functional neurological disorder. The healthy controls (green dots) were classified into the normative patterns of attachment, and the children with functional neurological disorder (including functional seizures) — the red dots — were classified into the at-risk patterns of attachment strategies. The rates of unresolved loss and trauma assessed via linguistic markers were 75% (n = 57/76) of children with functional neurological disorder versus 12% (n = 9/76) of controls. The Dynamic Maturational Model depicting patterns of attachment is reproduced with permission of Patricia Crittenden, © Patricia M. Crittenden, 2001.

Dysregulation of the Cortisol Awakening Response (a Product of HPA-Axis Function)

The hypothalamic-pituitary-adrenal axis is involved in the child's response to stress. Its end product, cortisol, is involved in energy regulation and in epigenetic programming — the biological embedding of experience — in the tissues (including the brain). In general, exposure to acute stress is associated with an increase in the cortisol awakening response (CAR), and chronic, prolonged, uncontrollable, or traumatic stress is associated with an attenuation of the CAR (Filaire et al., 2013). Children and adolescents with FND (13 of 32, or 41%, with functional seizures) showed the latter pattern (Chung et al., 2022). One FND subgroup showed an attenuated CAR and another showed a reversed CAR (attenuation to the point of reversal). See Figure A.4. On self-report — using the Early Life Stress Questionnaire (ELSQ) — children and adolescents with FND reported significantly more adverse childhood experiences (ACEs). This finding of increased ACEs has been found across different cohorts.

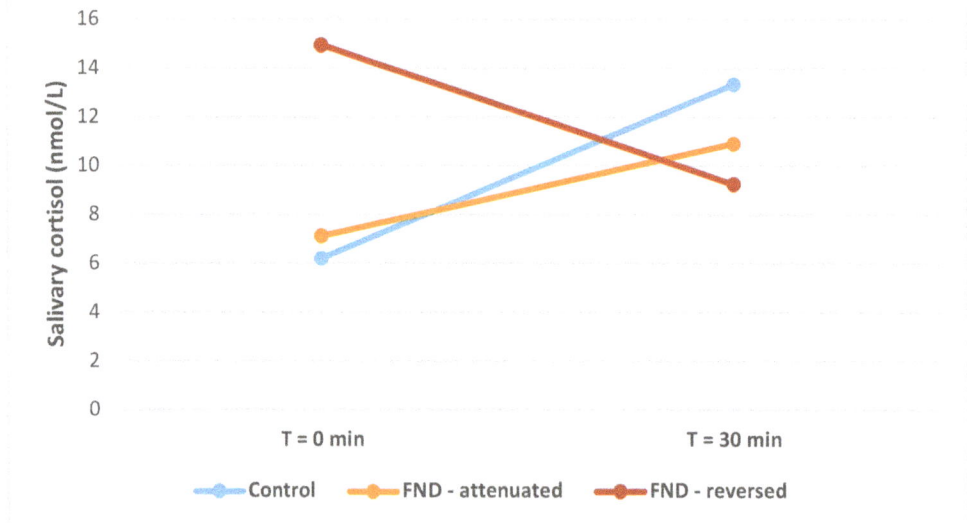

Figure A.4 Cortisol awakening response in children with functional neurological disorder. Visual depiction of the cortisol awakening response in children with functional neurological disorder and healthy controls. One subset of children with functional neurological disorder had an attenuated cortisol awakening response, and another had a reversed cortisol awakening responses, suggesting significant dysregulation of the HPA axis. © Kasia Kozlowska 2022

Increased Activation of the Autonomic Nervous System

Two research studies from our Mind-Body Program — from which 29/56 (51%) and 31/98 (32%) of participants had functional seizures — have shown that children and adolescents with FND show increased autonomic arousal in the resting state: elevated heart rate, increased skin conductance, and decreased heart rate variability) (Chudleigh et al., 2019; Kozlowska, Palmer, et al., 2015). See Figure A.5. These measures show that their autonomic nervous systems are in an activated state — are switched on more than they should be.

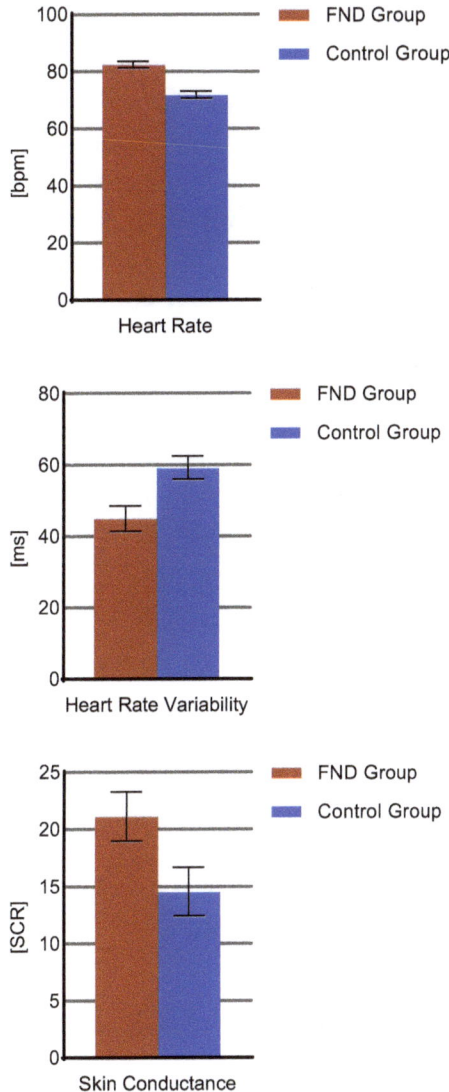

Figure A.5 Autonomic nervous system activation in children with functional neurological disorder. The bar charts show differences in resting-state heart rate (in beats per minute), heart rate variability (in milliseconds), and skin conductance (number of peaks in the SCR data) between children with functional neurological disorder and healthy controls.
© Kasia Kozlowska 2022

197

Increased Cortical Arousal and Role of Hyperventilation

In collaboration with other researchers, our mind-body team was able to use the electroencephalogram (EEG) to look at brain function in children and adolescents with FND (including functional seizures). One study extracted event-related potentials (ERPs) from the EEG to look at cortical (brain) arousal. This study showed that children and adolescents with FND (32 of 56, or 57%, with functional seizures) showed a more robust response to a sound stimulus — greater activation — than healthy controls (Kozlowska, Melkonian, et al., 2017). Another study measured power from different frequency ranges. This study showed that children and adolescents with functional seizures (vs. healthy controls) had more activation in the high-frequency power bands (beta and gamma) in the resting state and that increases in network metrics (beta and gamma power bands) correlated with autonomic system arousal (Radmanesh et al., 2020). Children with FND but no functional seizures also showed increased arousal, though the level was lower than in children and adolescents with functional seizures and higher than in healthy controls. A more recent study (using a hyperventilation task) from our colleagues in Canada — from Alberta Children's Hospital — showed that children and adolescents with functional seizures maintained activation in the beta power band (a high-frequency band) following hyperventilation (Braun et al., 2021), whereas healthy controls were able to down-regulate back to baseline. Hyperventilation is known to increase cortical arousal, which should settle when the child or adolescent stops hyperventilating. That is, the arousal should not persist, as it does in children and adolescents with functional seizures.

Separate from a hyperventilation task under laboratory conditions, in real life many children and adolescents with functional seizures hyperventilate in response to stress. Along these lines, in a clinical study of children and adolescents experiencing functional seizures, our Mind-Body Program found that hyperventilation triggered seizures in over 50% of the children and adolescents in the sample (32/60; 53%) (Kozlowska, Rampersad, et al., 2017). Our colleagues from Canada have likewise found that managing hyperventilation is important in the treatment of children and adolescents with functional seizures (Sawchuk et al., 2020a, 2020b).

Emotion Processing in Children with FND

In a research study from our Mind-Body Program, we found that children and adolescents with FND (29 of 57, or 51%, with functional seizures) had faster reaction times to emotion faces than healthy controls. See Figure A.6. This result indicates that children and adolescents with FND allocate more resources to emotion stimuli — in this instance, emotion faces — than healthy controls, presumably as a means of checking the environment for the presence of threat (Kozlowska et al., 2013).

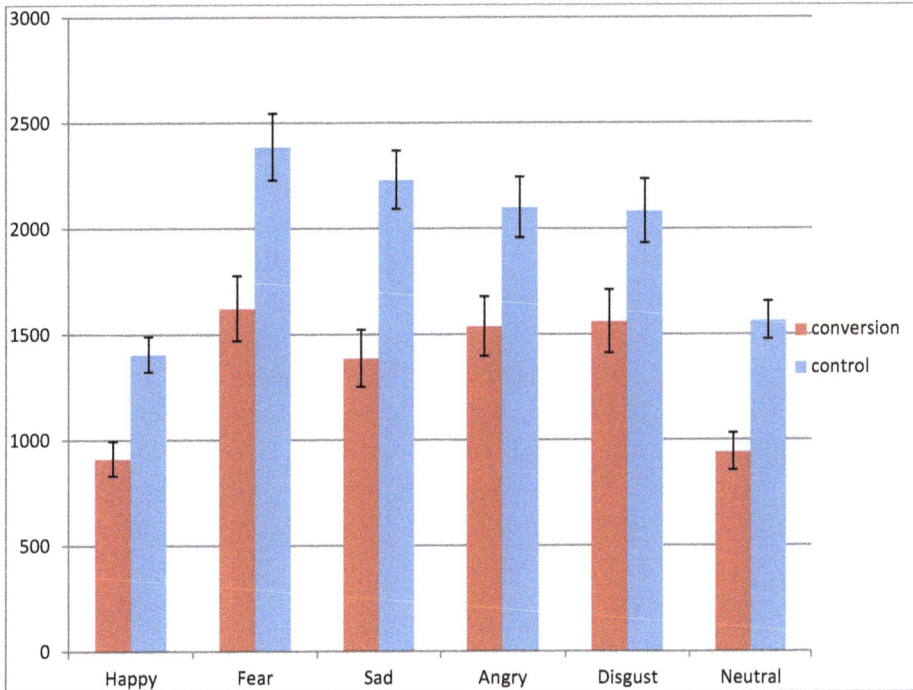

Figure A.6 Faster reaction times to emotion faces in children with functional neurological disorder. Reaction times to emotion faces for children and adolescents with functional neurological disorder and healthy controls. © Kasia Kozlowska 2016

Brain-Imaging Research

In another study from our Mind-Body Program, a group of children and adolescents with FND (12 of 25, or 48%, with functional seizures) participated in a small study using magnetic resonance imaging (MRI) (Kozlowska, Griffiths, et al., 2017). One key finding was increased grey matter volumes in the left supplementary motor area (SMA). The SMA — which lies in the dorsomedial frontal cortex, at the interface of motor and emotion processing — is involved in multiple motor- and emotion-processing functions. The study also found a correlation between increased SMA volumes and faster reaction times in identifying emotions on the study's face-recognition task. These findings suggest that the previous experiences of these children and adolescents not only affected their behavioural responses to emotion faces but also resulted in plasticity changes in the brain — that is, the biological embedding of experience (Boyce et al., 2021; Nelson, 2013).

Another group of children and adolescents with FND (13 of 31, or 42%, with functional seizures) participated in our Mind-Body Program's resting-state study, in which we used a new methodology called *independent component analysis* (ICA) (Rai et al., 2022). ICA is a computer-driven approach that is helpful for looking at brain function in a more holistic way: from the perspective of neural networks and the relationships between them. This study identified eight networks that showed differences in neural network function — in particular, increased or decreased connectivity to key brain regions — in children with FND. In one region, the frontoparietal network, which is involved in cognitive-control functions, the aberrant changes (decreased connectivity with the insula) were more pronounced in children and adolescents with functional seizures than in children with FND but no functional seizures. This result suggests more extensive neural network changes in children and adolescents with functional seizures — changes that potentially have the following consequences: more difficulties regulating arousal; more difficulties in regulating emotions and illness-promoting cognitions; and increased vulnerability to neural network dysregulation, potentially manifesting as functional seizures.

In a current study, not yet reported, we also examined their neurochemical brain profiles using MRI spectroscopy. The data from this study will be out shortly.

Key Messages from the Emerging Research Base

Children and adolescents with FND report or show the following:

- Increased numbers of adverse childhood experiences (ACEs) during their lifespans
- Increased body (autonomic) and brain arousal in the resting state—that is, a state of activation at baseline
- Increased reactivity to stress (emotional stimuli, auditory stimuli, or hyperventilation)
- Functional MRI findings of aberrant changes in resting-state neural network function, with increased vulnerability to neural network dysregulation, potentially manifesting as functional seizures
- Structural MRI findings of probable plasticity changes

A Hypothetical Aetiological Model

In view of the above-described research findings, and also a growing body of research from the adult literature, we can hypothesise that the neurobiology of FND (including functional seizures) involves a complex relationship between adverse childhood experiences, dysregulated neurophysiological, emotional, and cognitive processes, and experience-dependent plasticity changes within the brain (see Figure A.7).

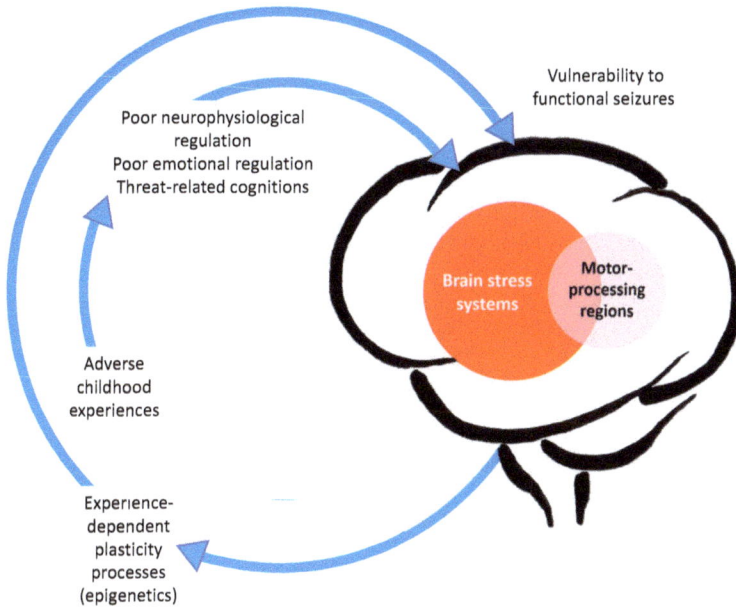

Figure A.7 The hypothetical aetiology of functional seizures. Visual representation linking adverse life experiences, stress-system activation, and epigenetic/plasticity processes that increase vulnerability for functional seizures (functional neurological disorder). © Kasia Kozlowska 2021

Functional Seizures: Fact Sheet

(for printing out)

The **Fact Sheet** on the following two pages is available as a free PDF file from the publisher. Scan the QR code below or type in your web browser: **https://www.australianacademicpress.com.au/page/55/Support_Materials** to go direct to the publisher's website Downloads page and then click on the download link for resources from this book. An email address is required to begin the download.

Please note. Translations of this Fact Sheet in several languages are also available for download.

FUNCTIONAL SEIZURES: FACT SHEET

WHAT ARE FUNCTIONAL SEIZURES?

Functional seizures are sudden, time-limited episodes of brain-network dysregulation that occur in the context of high arousal. Arousal—in the brain and body—refers to the level of activation. When the young person's brain and body are calm, the level of arousal is low. When the young person's brain and body activate in response to the challenges of daily living, arousal increases. In the normal course of events, arousal increases in response to a challenge—to enable the young person to meet that challenge —and then decreases (down-regulates) back to baseline. But young people with functional seizures activate their systems—including brain networks—into a state of overdrive and temporary dysregulation.

There are a number of different ways that a functional seizure might look. A young person might experience a loss of voluntary control of motor function, including shaking, jerking, twitching, loss of movement, or falling down. The young person can also experience a change in consciousness—or even loss of consciousness— including zoning out, feeling weird or disconnected, being unresponsive, difficulty thinking clearly, or slumping down. Functional seizures can also change in their presentation over time.

Functional seizures are different from epileptic seizures. Epileptic seizures are caused by sudden, abnormal electrical discharges in the brain. Functional seizures can look just like epileptic seizures, but they are not caused by abnormal electrical discharges. Instead, they arise in the context of chronic or severe stress that affects the functioning of the brain. These stressors including the following: (1) physical stressors such as pain, hyperventilation, illness, or fatigue; (2) emotional stressors such as grief, worry, distressing memories, or sudden fear or anxiety; (3) relational stressors such as difficulties in peer or family relationships; (4) academic stress such as pending exams, difficulty keeping up with classwork, or expectations of high academic achievement; and (5) a combination of these. Unlike epileptic seizures, which can be dangerous, functional seizures are not dangerous.

Although many people have never heard of functional seizures, they are quite common; studies suggest that up to a third of the seizure presentations to neurology departments are functional seizures.

A diagnosis of functional seizures will be made by your neurologist based on information that may include your clinical history, witnessed descriptions, home videos, a video electroencephalogram (vEEG), and any other necessary medical tests.

WHAT IS THE TREATMENT FOR FUNCTIONAL SEIZURES?

Functional seizures respond well to treatment, and most young people—with the help of their families— successfully learn how to manage them.

OTHER NAMES FOR FUNCTIONAL SEIZURES . . .

Functional seizures are a subtype of Functional Neurological Symptom Disorder (FND). There are many other names used for functional seizures:

- Stress seizures
- Non-epileptic seizures
- Non-epileptic attacks
- Pseudoseizures
- Psychogenic seizures
- Psychogenic non-epileptic seizures
- Dissociative seizures
- Dissociative attacks
- Dissociative non-epileptic seizures

Before treatment can begin, the young person, family, and treating team will work together to understand what might be triggering and maintaining the seizures. Because the life experiences and challenges of all young people are unique to them and their families, the origins, triggers, and maintaining factors will be different for each young person.

Treatment usually involves the following components:

- *Mind-body regulation strategies:* The young person uses these strategies to manage and, over time, to prevent the functional seizures. Mind-body strategies include interventions such as slow breathing, grounding approaches, mindfulness, visualisation, and progressive muscle relaxation.

- *Medication:* There is no specific medication for treating functional seizures. Medication may be prescribed (1) to reduce the high levels of arousal in the body that make the young person prone to the functional seizures and that undercut the capacity to learn other mind-body strategies for managing the functional seizures, (2) to treat anxiety or depression, which often coexist with functional seizures, or (3) to help with sleep. Functional seizures are more resistant to treatment if comorbid anxiety or depression and poor sleeping are not addressed.

- *Regular family meetings:* The family supports the young person to implement the treatment in the home setting, and the family works in collaboration with the treatment team to address other physical, emotional, or relational stressors in the young person's life and in the family context.

- *Physiotherapy* aims to promote positive expectations for the young person's physical wellbeing and to build physical and emotional resilience. Physiotherapists will design a progressive program that helps restore and optimise body strength, fitness, resilience, and physical function.

- *School intervention:* The young person's school may need support to manage the functional seizures when they occur at school. The school may also need to address stressors in the school environment (e.g., bullying, learning difficulties, or problems with peers) or to implement a reintegration program if the young person has not been attending regularly.

HOW SHOULD FUNCTIONAL SEIZURES BE MANAGED?

While the young person is learning to manage the functional seizures, the episodes will continue to occur. However, over the course of treatment, the frequency and intensity of the functional seizures will decrease. The young person, family, school, and treating team need to work together to develop a plan for managing functional seizures. The following information should be kept in mind:

- Functional seizures are not dangerous; calling an ambulance is not necessary. Instead, the young person, family, and school will implement a management plan for functional seizures.

- After learning to read his/her body, the young person will become adept at picking up the warning signs that a functional seizure might occur. The young person will then practice moving to a safe position (e.g., onto the floor or a bean bag) and implement the mind-body strategies that he/she has learnt for managing or preventing the episodes.

- Over time, as the young person practices the self-regulation strategies, he/she will become increasingly able to calm his/her body to avert the functional seizures.

- The young person is the only person who can manage his/her own body. Parents and teachers need to step back and give the young person space to implement the regulation strategies. The responsible adult needs to stay calm. Generally, only one adult needs to oversee the young person during the functional seizure—which can be done quietly, from a distance. A lot of attention and fussing over the young person will not help. In fact, research suggests that attention can increase the frequency and duration of functional seizures. Likewise, a state of high arousal is contagious. So, if the responsible adult is unable to stay calm, the young person's state of heightened arousal will increase further, making it even more difficult for him/her to settle down.

- If the young person experiences a functional seizure, he/she needs to assume, or the responsible adult needs to help him/her move to, a safe position. The responsible adult will then need to wait until the functional seizure has reached a natural end.

- When the functional seizure is over, the young person can return to the activity that he/she was engaged in before the seizure started. Headaches or feelings of fatigue are common (significant energy has been expended).

Five-Step Plan
(pertaining to the young person)

(for printing out)

The **Five-Step Plan** on the following page is available as a free PDF file from the publisher. Scan the QR code below or type in your web browser:
https://www.australianacademicpress.com.au/page/55/Support_Materials
to go direct to the publisher's website Downloads page and then click on the download link for resources from this book. An email address is required to begin the download.

Please note. Translations of this Five-Step Plan in several languages are also available for download.

Pertaining to the young person

Step 1	Identify warning signs
Step 2	Make yourself safe (sit down or lie down)
Step 3	Implement a mind-body regulation strategy to calm your body (and brain) to avert the functional seizure
Step 4	Ride it out (if the functional seizure was not averted)
Step 5	Implement a mind-body regulation strategy to calm your body (and brain) once the functional seizure is over

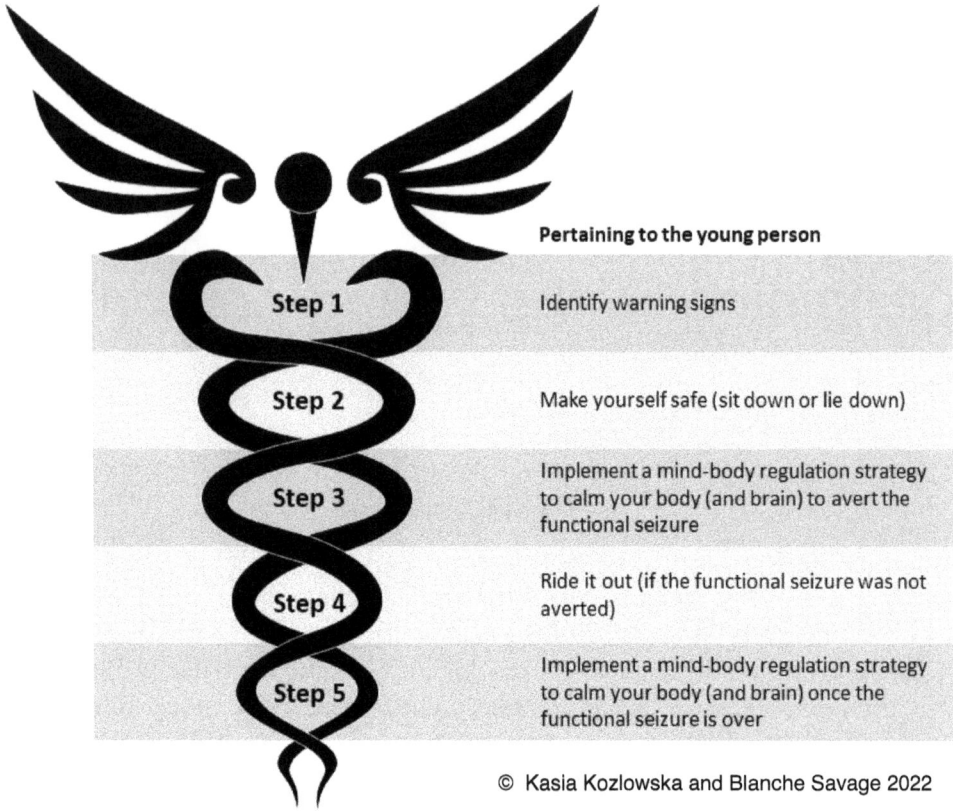

© Kasia Kozlowska and Blanche Savage 2022

Five-Step Plan
(pertaining to both the young person and parent [or other adult])

(for printing out)

The **Five-Step Plan — Parent** on the following page is available as a free PDF file from the publisher. Scan the QR code below or type in your web browser: **https://www.australianacademicpress.com.au/page/55/Support_Materials** to go direct to the publisher's website Downloads page and then click on the download link for resources from this book. An email address is required to begin the download.

Please note. Translations of this Five-Step Plan in several languages are also available for download.

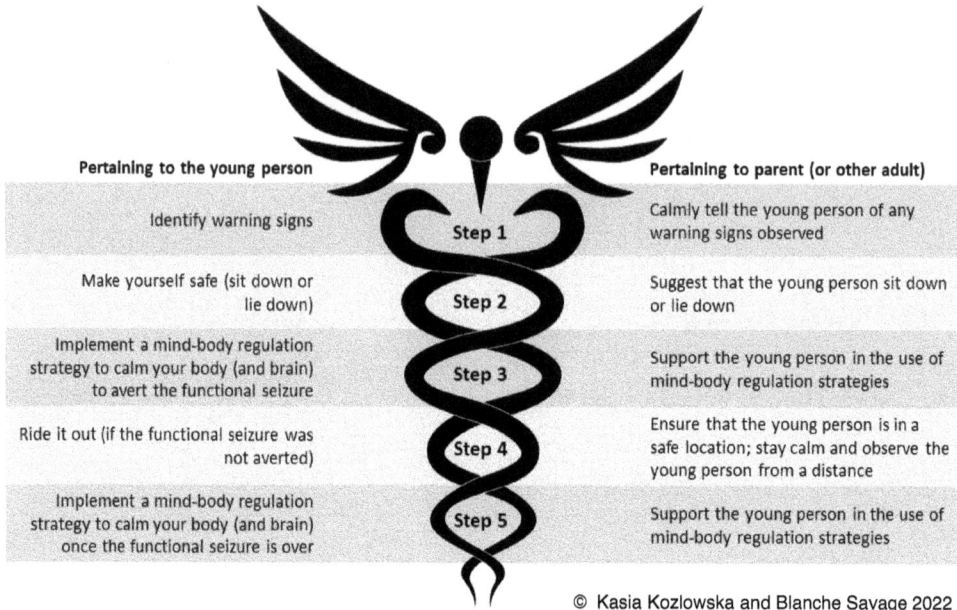

Pertaining to the young person		Pertaining to parent (or other adult)
Identify warning signs	**Step 1**	Calmly tell the young person of any warning signs observed
Make yourself safe (sit down or lie down)	**Step 2**	Suggest that the young person sit down or lie down
Implement a mind-body regulation strategy to calm your body (and brain) to avert the functional seizure	**Step 3**	Support the young person in the use of mind-body regulation strategies
Ride it out (if the functional seizure was not averted)	**Step 4**	Ensure that the young person is in a safe location; stay calm and observe the young person from a distance
Implement a mind-body regulation strategy to calm your body (and brain) once the functional seizure is over	**Step 5**	Support the young person in the use of mind-body regulation strategies

© Kasia Kozlowska and Blanche Savage 2022

Body Map (blank outline)

(for printing out)

The **Body Map** on the following page is available as a free PDF file from the publisher. Scan the QR code below or type in your web browser:
https://www.australianacademicpress.com.au/page/55/Support_Materials
to go direct to the publisher's website Downloads page and then click on the download link for resources from this book. An email address is required to begin the download.

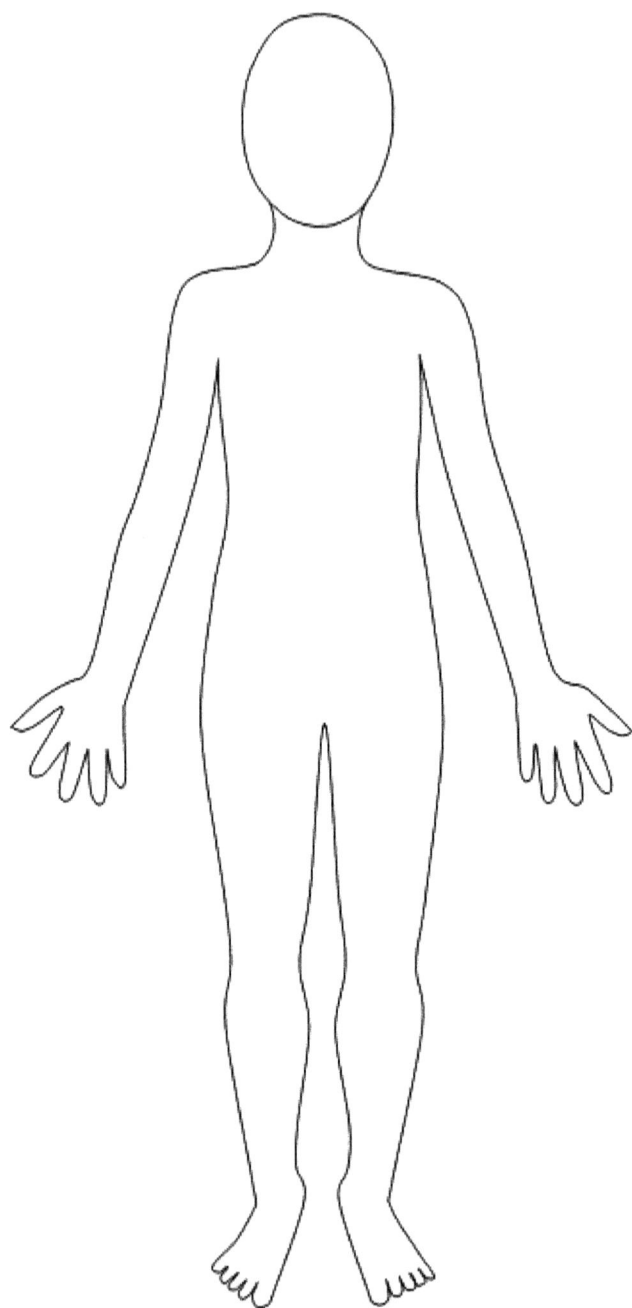

Traffic Light Safety Plan (blank, in black and white)

(for printing out)

The **Traffic Light Safety Plan** on the following page is available as a free PDF file from the publisher. Scan the QR code below or type in your web browser: **https://www.australianacademicpress.com.au/page/55/Support_Materials** to go direct to the publisher's website Downloads page and then click on the download link for resources from this book. An email address is required to begin the download.

Traffic Light Safety Plan for Managing Functional Seizures

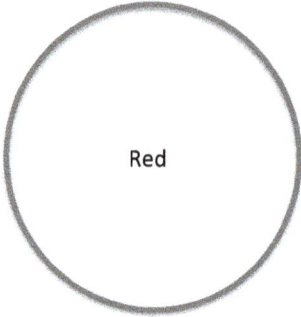

Signs:
-
-
-
-

Strategies:
-
-
-
-

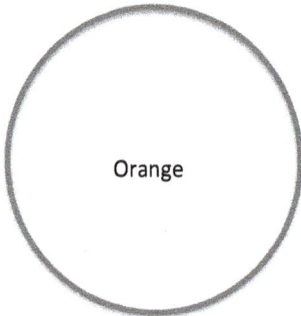

Signs:
-
-
-
-

Strategies:
-
-
-
-

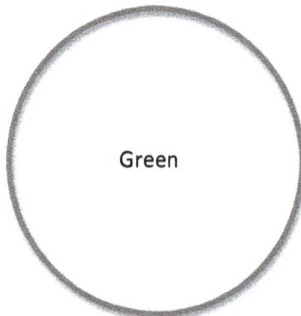

Signs:
-
-
-
-

Strategies:
-
-
-
-

Traffic Light Safety Plan (blank, in colour)

(for printing out)

The **Traffic Light Safety Plan — Colour** on the following page is available as a free PDF file from the publisher. Scan the QR code below or type in your web browser:
https://www.australianacademicpress.com.au/page/55/Support_Materials
to go direct to the publisher's website Downloads page and then click on the download link for resources from this book. An email address is required to begin the download.

Traffic Light Safety Plan for
Managing Functional Seizures

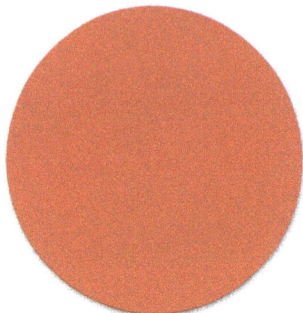

Signs:
-
-
-
-

Strategies:
-
-
-
-

Signs:
-
-
-
-

Strategies:
-
-
-
-

Signs:
-
-
-
-

Strategies:
-
-
-
-

Flowchart of Therapeutic Process

(for printing out)

The **Flowchart of Therapeutic Process** on the following page is available as a free PDF file from the publisher. Scan the QR code below or type in your web browser:

https://www.australianacademicpress.com.au/page/55/Support_Materials

to go direct to the publisher's website Downloads page and then click on the download link for resources from this book. An email address is required to begin the download.

Flowchart of Therapeutic Process

Referral triage by the mental health clinician (check that the following have been completed)

- A comprehensive medical assessment has been completed by a medical practitioner: physical examination, blood panel, and EEG (video EEG or EEG with review of video material by a paediatric neurologist).
- The medical practitioner has provided a positive diagnosis.
- The medical practitioner has provided an explanation.
- The young person and their family understand and accept the diagnosis.

Biopsychosocial assessment with the young person and the family

- The biopsychosocial assessment is to bring to light the young person's developmental history in the context of the family story, including a timeline of physical, psychological, and relational stressors (the story of the family and the story of the symptoms).
- The biopsychosocial assessment allows the clinician, the young person, and family to co-construct a formulation—a summary of predisposing, precipitating, and perpetuating factors.
- The formulation is used, in turn, to develop a treatment plan and to guide the treatment process.
- The young person and family need to understand the rationale for the treatment plan and to agree to (contract) to the treatment intervention (including the offered time frame).

Psychoeducation

- The initial psychoeducation intervention is delivered at the end of the biopsychosocial assessment. The clinician explains functional seizures again. The clinician also provides information about the treatment components and their rationale.
- Psychoeducation is usually repeated during, and integrated into, some of the early treatment sessions.

The mind-body treatment intervention with the mental health clinician and multidisciplinary team

Daily timetable	Five-Step Plan for Managing Functional Seizures	Daily pleasurable exercise or physiotherapy	Working with the family	Working with the school	Medications	Longer-term individual or family therapy
• Stabilise rhythms of daily living • Document daily practice of treatment elements	• Identify warning signs • Make yourself safe • Implement mind-body regulation strategy • Ride it out • Implement mind-body regulation strategy	• As a physical regulation strategy • To address deconditioning • To build resilience • For neuroprotection • To manage pain • To help sleep	• To address focus-of-attention • To hold positive expectations • To address family issues that contribute to the presentation	• Develop a school-based health care plan for managing functional seizures in the school setting • Implement integration of young person back to school	• To help decrease arousal • To help with sleep • For comorbid anxiety or depression • For comorbid functional gut disorders	• To work on issues not addressed by the Five-Step Plan intervention • To treat comorbid mental health disorders • To engage in a trauma-processing intervention • Ongoing family, parenting, or marital work (with parents)

Taking the mind-body intervention home

The family continues to implement all components of the mind-body intervention (as relevant to their particular context).